Praise for Claudine Wolk's

It Gets Easier!
...and Other Lies We Tell New Mothers

· ·

"The author does a brilliant job making her book stand out amidst the plethora of parenting books available to new moms. Her title says it all. There are so many myths associated with motherhood and so many feelings of guilt that often follow suit. But the author reassures you that you are not alone and does it all with levity and wit. Her examination of the stay-at-home mom versus the mom who works outside the home is wonderful. I really connected with Claudine, and I can't wait to see more books from her!"

—Tara Kompare,
author of *The Colic Chronicles*

"Fresh! Practical! Down-to-earth! If that's the kind of mothering advice you'd like, read this book. Claudine Wolk has thrown out the old wives' tales and gathered the best helpful hints on topics you really want to know about."

—Suzanne Zoglio, Ph.D., psychologist,
author of *Create a Life That Tickles Your Soul*

"*It Gets Easier . . . and Other Lies We Tell New Mothers* gives new moms uncensored advice they won't find anywhere else. Claudine tells it like it really is, with honesty and humor! Any one of her tips could save you hours of hassle or even cut down on sleepless nights for you and your baby."

—Amy Tiemann, Ph.D., psychologist,
author of the award-winning
Mojo Mom: Nurturing Your Self While Raising a Family
and creator of MojoMom.com

"Any time women, especially mothers, talk to one another honestly about their experiences, there's powerful good to be gained. Here, Claudine Wolk has done just that. My hat's off to her."

—Kate Fratti, columnist,
Bucks County Courier Times

"It's the perfect book for that new mom (or soon-to-be mom) about the pitfalls and obstacles that every mother inevitably confronts, and Wolk, in an empathetic, light-hearted, and most importantly, optimistic way, has written a guide that lets mom's know that it's going to be okay. The information provided by Wolk is invaluable. *It Gets Easier!* . . . also does a fantastic job of instilling confidence in moms everywhere."

—Jennifer Teaford,
Doylestown Bookstore, events coordinator

"*It Gets Easier!* . . . is a great read—great information in a quick and easy and very funny presentation."

—Dr. Leslie Frankel, OB/GYN,
Abington Hospital, Abington, PA

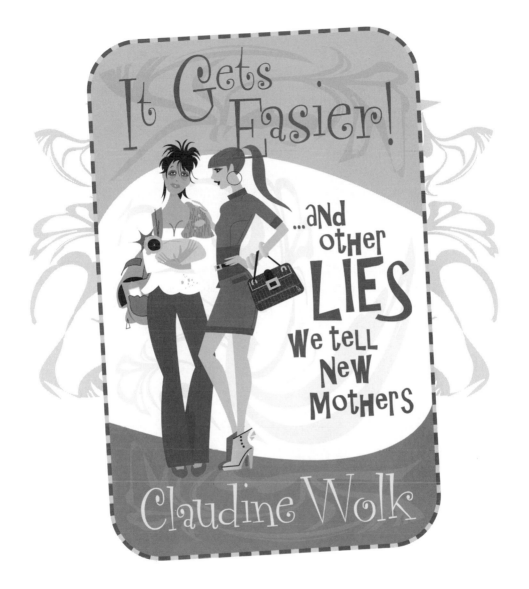

It Gets Easier!

...aNd other LIES We teLL NeW MotHers

Claudine Wolk

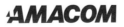

American Management Association

New York • Atlanta • Brussels • Chicago • Mexico City • San Francisco
Shanghai • Tokyo • Toronto • Washington, D.C.

Special discounts on bulk quantities of AMACOM books are available to corporations, professional associations, and other organizations. For details, contact Special Sales Department, AMACOM, a division of American Management Association, 1601 Broadway, New York, NY 10019. Tel: 212-903-8316. Fax: 212-903-8083.
E-mail: specialsls@amanet.org
Website: www.amacombooks.org/go/specialsales
To view all AMACOM titles go to: www.amacombooks.org

This publication is designed to provide accurate and authoritative information in regard to the subject matter covered. It is sold with the understanding that the publisher is not engaged in rendering legal, accounting, or other professional service. If legal advice or other expert assistance is required, the services of a competent professional person should be sought.

Library of Congress Cataloging-in-Publication Data

Wolk, Claudine.
  It gets easier! — and other lies we tell new mothers : a fun, practical guide to becoming a mom / Clauding Wolk.
      p. cm.
  Includes bibliographical references and index.
  ISBN 978-0-8144-1502-3
1. Mothers—Life sills guides.   2. Childbirth.   3. Infants—Care.
4. Motherhood—Humor.   I. Title.

HQ759.W5845 2009
649' .10852—DC22

                                            2009004736

Printing number

10 9 8 7 6 5 4 3 2 1

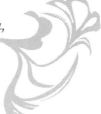

For Joseph, Casey, and Alyssa,
and for Joe,
my best friend.

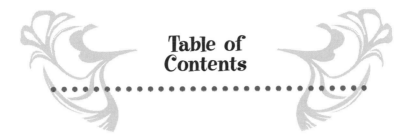

Table of Contents

Every effort has been made to ensure that the information contained in this book is complete and accurate. However, neither the publisher nor the author is engaged in rendering professional advice or services to the individual reader. The ideas, procedures, and suggestions contained in this book are not intended as a substitute for consulting your healthcare provider. All matters regarding the health of you and your baby require medical supervision. Neither the publisher nor the authors shall be liable or responsible for any loss or damage allegedly arising from any information or suggestions in this book.

—Claudine Wolk

Foreword

Of all the challenges that await you as a new mum, there is none as scary as the ghost of The Good Mommy — she of the slightly staring eyes and permanent-press smile. The Good Mommy is the spirit that dwells within us, whispering that we are doing it wrong, that we are screwing it up, that we are alone in what we feel.

The good news is that her haunting days are numbered, thanks to the work of fearless, funny, and forthright women like Claudine Wolk, and books like *It Gets Easier! ...And Other Lies We Tell New Mothers.*

When you bring a new baby into your life, what you need more than diapers and breastpumps is a girlfriend who's been there before, who's lived — and laughed — to tell the tale. And that goes double if it's a girlfriend who is 100 percent committed to telling you the truth (without the sugar-coating of the latest theory or hottest trend).

Claudine Wolk is that girlfriend. And that's what makes this book like a long, cool glass of iced tea on a sweltering summer day — or an ice pack on your post-partum stitches.

There are a thousand ways to be a great mother, which is both comforting and, at times, pretty confusing. Claudine helps you through the early motherhood maze by marking the major sign-posts, which many of the rest of us have had to stumble upon.

And she gives the lie, bless her, to the mythology that there are no rules when it comes to infant care. There are, in fact. And learning what they are and how to respect them may not exactly set you free — you'll need two to five decades more for that — but it will help you get the self-care you need to keep loving your life.

My own first baby turned 18 this year, so these days my broken sleep is more about how she's getting back from last night's party. Now I worry when she *doesn't* wake me up at 2 A.M.!

No, it doesn't get easier. But it does get different — the sorrows more complex, and the joys more multi-hued. But then we didn't decide to become mothers because it was easy. We did it because we thrive on challenge, on adventure. And this is life's biggest adventure — no matter how strenuously The Good Mommy tries to cut it down to size.

Hey. Maybe *that's* why there are no operating instructions — because parenthood is nothing whatsoever like a machine. There are only guidebooks because parenthood is very much like a journey.

Toss this one in your backpack. I guarantee it'll lighten your load.

Susan Maushart
Author of *The Mask of Motherhood,*
Wifework, and *What Women Want Next*

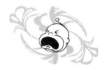

Preface

When I started this project, I was going to write what I called the comprehensive guide for the new mother. The book was going to cover all topics relating to motherhood: pregnancy, labor and delivery, recovery, and surviving being at home. I began writing this book when my firstborn son was a baby. That was fourteen years ago. At that time I had looked for a manual to help prepare me for motherhood and all that it entails. I couldn't find it. Of course, these days there are thousands of books available on the subject.

As I wrote mine, I tended to spend more time on some topics than on others. It turned out that I wasn't interested in writing the comprehensive guide after all. I felt that I had some great tips for being in the hospital and tips for labor and delivery, but I seemed to spend more time on what happens *after* you have a baby. As I wrote more, I tended to write about the "motherhood experience," and specifically as it relates to women of my generation.

I do not presume to speak for all women. We each have different thoughts and feelings regarding this experience we call motherhood. The fact remains, though, that much about caring for babies has not changed. Taking care of a baby these days is not very different from taking care of one years ago. Taking care of school-aged children is another matter; that is very different. The women of my generation needed solutions — and I realized that I wanted at least some of those solutions to come from the women who've successfully done this before us.

The "baby" topics I've covered are the ones that seem most essential to me: scheduling, getting the baby to sleep through the night, and dealing with the negative feelings about mothering that so few people talk about. The other baby-related discussion topics are all the nitty-gritty practical tips for the hospital and making it through those first few months. These are all the tips I wished I'd been fully equipped with before I ever made my first trip to a delivery room.

This experience of motherhood can be a lonely one. Women are afraid to broach many of the subjects on their minds for fear of being labeled a "bad" mother. Feeding on demand. Negative feelings about the new baby. Lack of sleep. Naptimes. Housework. To work or not to work? It can all prove overwhelming.

What women today want the most, I believe, is answers. This generation of mothers is so busy that they want to know what works and they are not afraid to try new things. New mothers want to flourish in their lives. Many may want to continue in their careers. All certainly want to continue to look and feel good, and they all want to continue to have good relationships with their spouses. I felt women needed a few tried and true tips and some direction to do more than survive this life stage called motherhood.

In order to uncover these tips, I interviewed hundreds of women and (some) men from the East Coast to the West Coast. I asked questions of anyone who would talk to me — friends and friends of friends, neighbors, family members, my mother, my mother-in-law, my mother's friends, women on playgrounds, and strangers on planes. Their insights as well as my personal experiences and research are in this book, along with a dash of humor — because we all know that humor can be that spoonful of sugar that makes the medicine go down, even if it is not easy.

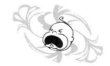

Acknowledgments

Most important, I thank my talented husband, Joe, for his never-ending creativity regarding the production of this book and for being my friend, lover, and partner, as well as a devoted father. Wow, Joe! I thank my father, Tom Feledick, my first editor, who taught me how to write with his insightful editing and unbelievable writing skills. I thank my mother, Peg Feledick, whose guidance, advice, insights and editing are threaded throughout this book. I thank my agent, Verna Dreisbach, for her unfailing perseverance in finding a terrific home for *It Gets Easier!* I thank the folks at AMACOM, particularly my editors, Ellen Kadin and Andy Ambraziejus, who believed in this project from the beginning and brought a great deal of heart to the production of the book. To Susan Maushart, whose belief in this book is the reason I kept writing it, and whose own popular books paved the way for "honesty in motherhood." I thank you.

I am grateful to Brian Taylor and Nina Taylor at Pneuma books and Sharon Castlen at Integrated Book Marketing. I am grateful to Lisa Henderling for her unbelievable cover design. I thank Chris Moyer for her artful cover design concept and Marge Brescia for her photography. I would also like to thank Judith Norkin who shared her writing talents with me. I am grateful to Heather Kelly, MA, IBCLC, who was nice enough to answer all of my questions about breastfeeding.

I am indebted to my friends, family, coworkers, neighbors, and strangers whom I met on playgrounds, on airplanes, in restaurants, and wherever I could find a mother or father who talked to me about being a new parent. I am most thankful to all the women writers who are gutsy enough to write about these issues. Every time I read their work I know that I am not alone in wanting to make motherhood a little easier for moms! Finally, I would like to acknowledge the members of my immediate family, who have encouraged me by their example to accomplish great things, including my grandmother, Marguerite, who would have gotten a kick out of this book; my Nana and Pop-pop, whose unconditional love I continue to feel; and my father-in-law, Joe, whose smile and laughter I miss every day.

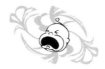

Chapter One

Insider Secrets!

Motherhood is the last thing I expected to be writing about when I graduated high school. Scholarship, scholarship, scholarship was all I could think about. When I got one to Saint Joseph's University in Philadelphia, I switched gears and focused on GPA, GPA, GPA. After graduating it became career, career, career. But after working for four years I found myself married and pregnant with my first child. It wasn't a long, thought-out decision. If I considered it at all, I thought, *You get married, you get pregnant.* Right? Right!

My son arrived in 1993, two weeks early. I was on my way out from work when my labor started. When I took him home from the hospital, I was about as uninformed as I could possibly be. I had read *What to Expect When You're Expecting*, of course, but I hadn't touched a childcare book. I figured taking care of my baby would just come to me and I would like it. I was wrong.

After about two weeks of feeding on demand (a.k.a. putting a bottle in my son's mouth every time he cried and my son not only eating poorly but screaming all the time)I was convinced he could not be mine and was ready to return him to the hospital. *How can women enjoy this?* I thought. "Liars, they're all liars," I told myself.

I scoured the bookshelves for help but found none. Not only did the books not cover this incessant crying or what to do about it, but they seemed to skip the truth about those first days and weeks altogether. I needed some answers, so I called the doctor. The doctor said he would grow out of it in about three months. Three months! What was I supposed to do for the next three months? Recreational drugs were not an option. I was sinking and sinking fast. I had gone from managing an accounting office of five professionals to holding, rocking, feeding, and changing a cranky infant. There was no smile on my face and not many on his either.

I could not believe this was motherhood: Misery and crying and being enslaved to a demanding infant. I was desperate for help. I needed the truth and I was willing to search for it wherever I could find it. Books didn't have it. Doctors were out. Finally I realized that other mothers would have the answers I was looking for. I started with my own.

"No one really likes it in the beginning," she confessed. Now she tells me. "It takes a little while to get that first smile and then you'll see it's all worth it."

It was a relief to discover that my own lack of happy feelings was normal, but I quickly moved on to more pressing matters.

"Demand feeding?" I asked. "I'm feeding this kid all the time and he still cries."

"I'm on it," she said. She spoke to a friend who let her in on "the schedule" and the rest is history. "The Schedule" was the first new mom "insider information" that I received in my quest for help. I discuss baby schedules in detail in Chapter Eight. Once I learned about the schedule, I suspected that there was more information out there to be discovered.

I was right. My continued research unearthed a treasure trove of tricks, secrets, and tips that mothers don't advertise. They remain tight-lipped because so much of what they have to say may not be considered politically correct. After all, who wants to actually admit that this experience of motherhood isn't always like the Ivory soap commercials?

Easy... I promise!

Some babies spit up a lot. It doesn't necessarily signify an allergy or an acid reflux problem. Sometimes what looks like a lot really isn't. Take a tablespoon of milk and spill it on the table and see how much it looks like.

The insider information was so helpful to me that I decided to record it so I could share it with other mothers. Survival, I felt, was all I was after. As the months passed and my son developed a reasonable schedule, I decided to research the other issues I was dealing with. That research took the form of informal discussions with other mothers working full-time outside the house. After two years, I decided to be an at-home mom. Here is where things started to get interesting. I had a whole new territory to explore. I began visiting the places stay-at-home moms go — shopping malls, indoor playgrounds, outdoor playgrounds, parks, schools, and preschools — and I spoke with anyone who would talk to me. The questions were generally the same:

* How much is too much spit up?
* Do you use a schedule?
* How many weeks do you think it is before a mom can expect her baby to sleep through the night?
* Do you let your baby cry?
* Do you feed cereal before the first year?

Easy... I promise!

Well-rested babies sleep better than poorly rested ones. Don't skip naps in order to help your baby sleep better at night. It will backfire!

I also loved to ask the "forbidden" questions, although I reserved those for mothers of older babies and children.

* How do you feel being at home?
* Do you miss work?
* Has your relationship with your husband changed?
* Why don't women talk about how they *really* feel?

For twelve years I recorded other women's thoughts and my personal experience with what really works. The learning spans three children, a move across country and back, and several forays into the workforce. This book is my best effort to provide new mothers with help in a humorous and honest voice — an alternative to the old adage, "It gets easier. I promise."

Of course, one of the most common sources of information on the subject of pregnancy and childrearing is books. I, too, read books in preparation for pregnancy and found their information useful; I still do. What I felt these books were lacking and what I have tried to provide for you is the uncensored advice. You know, the "behind the scenes" advice that no one ever tells us. This is the kind of counsel I was desperately searching for on the bookshelf and ended up finding by talking to other mothers — those from my generation and from past generations. I am excited to share it all with you because I honestly believe it will help tremendously in your efforts to take care of your new baby and to take care of yourself and your family in the twenty-first century. It will at least give you a leg-up on the experience.

Summary

It was a bit disconcerting to realize that new motherhood was not quite as easy as I thought it was going to be. I was always looking over my shoulder, wondering if anyone could tell that I didn't actually like motherhood every second of the day. The truth is, although many will never admit it, new motherhood is incredibly tough. It is back-breaking, neverending, confusing, frustrating, and largely thankless. Aren't you glad you decided to read this book? I sure know how to spread the sunshine around, don't I? The good news is — help is here. Read on to uncover some great advice from research and experience that will open the door to the truth about motherhood and the ways to make it a bit easier. Taking some of this advice to heart will enable you to actually enjoy motherhood a whole lot more *without* your having to lie about how you really feel.

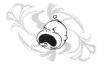

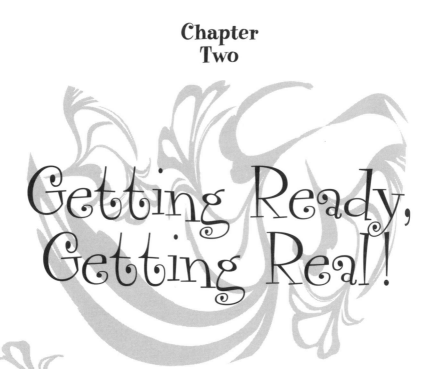

Chapter
Two

Getting Ready,
Getting Real!

It's strange how everyone keeps the truly helpful advice to themselves when you're pregnant because a pregnant woman receives no shortage of unhelpful and unwelcome advice. The source of that is usually strangers who mistakenly believe that your pregnant body is public property. When I was eight months pregnant with my first child, I had a woman stop me in the mall and tell me that I shouldn't be drinking diet cola. For some reason when it comes to a pregnant woman, all etiquette flies out the window and everyone seems to have something to say.

Ignoring "advice" from random strangers is probably a good idea — especially when it comes with a dash of judgment or negativity. Another good thing to ignore is everyone's scary stories. You know the kind. The "I was in labor for ten days and I only dilated to three centimeters" kind. Ignore them. You probably shouldn't even dwell too much on the "scary" chapters in books. Years ago our mothers didn't even have access to this information. I wonder sometimes if it's better to go into the situation a little less knowledgeable of all the things that could possibly go wrong. Did I say *scary*? Did I say *things that could go wrong*? Forget about that. Let's focus on before-birth preparations — and I don't mean preparing a fancy nursery. I'm talking about the advice you really need that no one tells you.

> **Easy... I promise!**
>
> **When you're getting up with the baby during the night, make sure you hold the banister as you carry the baby down the stairs.**

Unnecessary Preparations
The "Birthing Plan"

After seeing close to a thousand episodes of *A Baby Story*, you may feel motivated to prepare a birthing plan. The nurses in the hospital just love these by the way. They have a good chuckle. The birthing plan is a step-by-step plan for the faultless delivery that will welcome little Kaitlyn or Noah into the world.

Most birth plans include these "essential" elements:

* Stay at home for as long as possible when labor begins.
* Play soothing music.
* Watch a video.
* Surround yourself with *all* your relatives.
* Refuse all drugs.
* Squirt the bundle of joy out while your husband feeds you ice chips and coaches you through your breathing.
* Celebrate with champagne after delivery.
* Fill out form for the most faultless delivery of the year.

In reality most women experience something like this:

* Feel total uncertainty about whether or not you are even in labor.
* Try to do the breathing/ice chip thing for about ten hours.
* Husband rubs your back for about ten minutes and then exclaims that his wrist hurts.
* The doctor checks your cervix and lets you know that after all that hard work, you're still only three centimeters dilated.
* The doctor breaks your water with something that looks like a knitting needle. Could that really be a medical instrument?
* Walk around or sit in a rocking chair.
* Listen to the amniotic fluid that continues to splash on the floor every so often.
* Climb back in bed and continue with your breathing as your husband and the doctor discuss the score of the sporting event that is on television.
* Realize that breathing does absolutely nothing for the pain, which ironically does not go away completely when the monitor shows the contraction is over.
* Beg for the anesthesiologist. Although the needle used to seem terrifying, it now appears as a beacon of salvation.
* Ignore your husband who reminds you that medication was not on the birthing plan.
* Dutifully explain that if you don't get the epidural you will perform a vasectomy on him yourself when you leave the hospital.
* Feel the almost instant relief from the epidural and swear that after this is over you are going to leave your husband for the anesthesiologist.

* Start pushing.
* Push for about an hour before the doctor decides that in addition to an episiotomy, he's going to use suction to retrieve your baby.
* The baby emerges with a conehead and pees on your husband.
* Ask the nurse to place your birthing plan in the trash can.
* Forget about the champagne and ask for a turkey sandwich instead.

It's okay if you want to have a birthing plan, but just put "Keep an open mind" at the top of the list. Births don't always go as planned. The important thing is that you survive the birth and go home with a healthy newborn. If the pain is greater than you expected, ask for an epidural. Be open to making some changes to your birthing plan as your labor progresses.

Necessary Preparations
To Medicate or Not to Medicate

The decision to use medication during labor will probably result in your first encounter with mother-guilt. If you're trying to make that important decision, watch out for unsolicited advice. "Try not to use medication. It's not good for the baby," most people say. Forget about that. The choice is yours. You are the one going through labor and delivering the baby. If you want to experience labor without medication, try it! However, do not feel guilty if you change your mind.

Most sources note that 95 percent of expectant mothers use epidurals. The medication is there for your use and it does not pose any threat to the baby. The American College of Obstetricians and Gynecology offers this view on the subject:

Labor results in severe pain for many women. There is no other circumstance where it is considered acceptable for a person to experience severe pain, amenable to safe intervention, while under a physician's care. Maternal request is a sufficient justification for pain relief during labor.[1]

Works for me! Where was this quote when I was having my first child?

Talk to your doctor about epidural procedure contingencies. Specifically, if your doctor is not available at the hospital when you are in labor, *find out who else can authorize the epidural for you.* A close friend of mine was told she could not receive the epidural because her doctor was not there to okay it. She had to go without. Ouch!

The most important thing about this momentous decision is this: The choice is yours, and you can always change your mind! Just give it some thought before you get into the delivery room.

Breast or Bottle?

If the decision to use medication during labor is a new mom's first test of mother-guilt, then the decision about whether to breast-feed is definitely her second. Everyone wants you to breast-feed. Your obstetrician, your pediatrician, society, LaLeche — everyone. As the saying goes, "Breastfeeding is best!" Here's the problem: None of those people are going to be with you at two in the morning when you are feeding your newborn for the twelfth time that day — or for any of the hours of any of the days for that matter.

Breastfeeding is a personal decision for a new mother; after all, it intimately involves her mammary glands. The vast majority of women I've interviewed who have tried it love breastfeeding and absolutely swear by it. But there are some women who have tried it and hated it. Those women report that they found it unfulfilling, physically draining, and painful.

What I've discovered (and you undoubtedly have to) is that there is no shortage of opinions on the subject. All the mom books have an opinion. Some try to talk you into it, and other books include the author's confessions and apologies for either not trying it or not sticking with it. In *Sippy Cups Are Not for Chardonnay*, Stephanie Wilder-Taylor describes how she lied to her postpartum doula, telling her she was continuing to breast-feed after she had given up and switched to bottles.[2] Imagine that, being afraid to tell the truth to the person you're paying to help you! Likewise, in *Baby Laughs*, Jenny McCarthy had me in stitches when I read her "sure-fire way" to get a "breast-nazi" out of your hospital room is to tell her that you just "shit the bed."[3]

Where does all this leave the new mom? Well, most importantly I would advise you to have an opinion before you get to the hospital. The hospital personnel will ask you right away if you are going to breast-feed because they'll want to start the process right away. If you are not quite sure by the time you go into labor, ask as many questions as you want and keep an open mind. If you are sure that you do not want to breast-feed, get your opinion out in the open early. Let everyone who asks know how you feel and state it with conviction.

When I had my first child, I was the first of my friends to get pregnant. Not only was I unaware of the breastfeeding versus bottle-feeding debate, I also hadn't read a thing or researched a thing about breastfeeding. I literally went from the business world to the "new mom" world with no stopping in between. I felt no guilt about feeding my firstborn with a bottle. I was going back to work and breastfeeding didn't seem like a long-term possibility. I didn't know many new mothers, so there was no one to give me a hard time about not breastfeeding.

When I had my third child seven years later, the breastfeeding landscape had changed dramatically. I planned to stick to what I knew — bottle-feeding — but I was definitely lobbied to try breastfeeding in the hospital. I found I had to be firm. I purposefully stated to anyone who would listen, "I'm bottle-feeding, thanks!" Finally, when my pediatrician entered my room for my baby's first check-up he said to me, "Do you realize that you are the only mother out of seventeen in our maternity ward who is *not* breastfeeding?" I did not; I hadn't been out of bed conducting a survey. Then he said something really surprising: "Good for you!" Interesting, huh?

I discuss breastfeeding tips and issues in more detail in Chapter Four. However, let me state here that I would fight for a mother to either breast-feed or bottle-feed. I feel strongly that if a mother wants to breast-feed she should do it and be able to do it at work, in the park, or anywhere in public for that matter. It cracks me up that a society that allows breasts to be shown on TV, in movies, on magazine covers, in Hooters, and just about everywhere else gets so offended when faced with a breastfeeding mother. I just don't get it. Give her all the support she needs, all the time she needs, all the freedom she needs to do it.

By the same token, leave those bottle-feeding women alone! It's obvious that many women use formula, either exclusively or as a supplement, at some point. After all, we never hear anything on the news about the formula companies going out of business. So let's come out of the closet.

Your concern as a new mom is to take care of your baby to the best of your ability. In order to do that you must first take care of yourself. If that means breastfeeding, terrific. If that means bottle-feeding, no worries!

The "Talk" with Your Husband

Before you give birth you'll have plenty of opportunities to say your husband's four favorite words: "We have to talk." Yep, that's right, you'll get to see the hairs on the back of his neck stand straight up as fear creeps down his spine.

Talk to your husband ahead of time about how things may be after the baby is born. Do not, I repeat, *do not* wait until after the baby is born to discuss these issues. That would be like waiting until after you get married to discuss whether you want to have children. You should also open a dialogue with your obstetrician and the pediatrician about some of these issues. They can be invaluable resources. Here's a list of the hot topics. As you can see, some will probably require more than one discussion to reach agreement.

* *If it's a boy, do we circumcise?* This is definitely *not* a question you want to ask for the first time in the hospital. It's also one your husband is sure to have an opinion on.

* *What does breastfeeding entail?* "Honey, heads-up. My breasts are going to be set free, all the time, and you may be denied access to them for a while, but enjoy watching your baby go at 'em."

* *Are we both going to continue working?* You might say this: "I would like to stop working as soon as possible, how are *you* going to make that happen for me?" Or maybe something like this: "There is no way I am going to quit my job. Have you ever thought about being a stay-at-home dad?

* *Who will care for the child during the day?* "Let's look for an Alice from the *Brady Bunch* type nanny rather than a young au pair from a foreign country."

* *How are we both going to get the child to and from daycare?* Discuss splitting the duty. You both made the baby; you should both participate in transporting the baby to daycare.

* *What household chores are we going to split up?* In other words, giving birth won't magically turn you into June Cleaver.

* *Who will get up in the middle of the night?* Just because you have the boobs doesn't mean you have to be up alone in the middle of the night. There is always pumping, or he could bring the baby to you, or maybe he could just keep you company. That will happen in a little world I like to call Every New Mother's Fantasy! If you're bottle-feeding, then boobs are irrelevant!

* *Who will do the grocery shopping?* You could always look into grocery store delivery, either online shopping and free delivery.

* *What kinds of dinners can we expect to make?* Let him know if you survived on take-out before the baby, you can do so now.

* *What to anticipate with Mom's recovery?* You might say something like this: "My recovery will be long and arduous. I cannot be expected to cook, clean, or do laundry. My sole activity will be to care for the baby and rest for at least a year." I didn't say it would work.

* *How long after can we resume sex?* "Sex will be an interesting activity to think about again...after a full year has passed or maybe in four short weeks! I just don't know. Please try to get the image of a baby coming out of my vagina out of your head. It might spoil the mood. And by the way, Yes, Virginia, you can get pregnant right away after having a baby, so if you want to get back in there, plan accordingly."

* *Are we going to have any visitors?* "Put a lock on the door, barricade it if you have to. No one gets past that front door unless they come bearing one of two things: food or cleaning products!"

* *Are we going to hire any help?* "Get out the Yellow Pages — we're going to need a bigger boat." (If you don't recognize that quote, you need to watch *Jaws* again.)

Practical Preparations
Stock Up on Maxi Pads

On a practical note, have a supply of maxi pads available. Your husband will definitely appreciate it if you shop for these ahead of time and don't have to send him out to the store. Don't laugh! No one told me I would need maxi pads after childbirth — and you may even need them before. If your water breaks at home (or heaven forbid, while you're out in public), you'll need them before you get to the hospital. When I went into labor with my second child my water broke in the middle of the night. I made it to the toilet and then sat on it as I called my doctor and my parents. On my way to the bathroom, I asked my husband to bring me some pads from the other bathroom where I had stored them. After I got off the phone I saw that he had left five tampons on the counter for me. "What am I going to do with these?" I asked. "Stack them up like Lincoln Logs?"

Pack Your Bag

Yes, this is an easy one, and it's a piece of advice you've probably heard. But let's talk about some not so obvious things to pack. One of the most helpful tips I can share is to have a new notebook and a pen with you to write down the number of feed-

Easy... I promise!

When the doctors and nurses advise you not to lift anything heavier than the baby, they mean it. Ignore this advice at your own peril!

ings and the number of wet/dirty diaper changes (noting the times for each). The notebook will also come in handy to jot down questions for the pediatrician, obstetrician, or nurses. You'll likely think of many things when you are alone but forget to ask when the doctors and nurses visit you and your baby. The notebook can also be used to jot down feelings and events that may occur during the day. My notebooks ended up being a source I could consult for a history of each baby.

Bring phone numbers of friends and family and any emergency numbers you may need. You should also bring your pediatrician's and obstetrician's. You don't know how much time you will have to call people before you go to the hospital, and with cell phones, you can reach anyone you'll want to call.

Bring your *What to Expect When You're Expecting* and *Dr. Spock's Baby and Childcare* (or any other baby books you're reading) in case you have an immediate question that you want to research. Keep them on your table by your bed so you can reach them easily postpartum.

Be sure to pack your comfy socks, a clip to pull back your hair, shampoo, facial soap, body soap, and a cosmetics case with the basics — moisturizer, mascara, and lipstick if you wear it. You'll feel more like yourself if you have these items with you.

Stash Some Pacifiers

I know you have probably already decided against using a "binky," but hide a supply of them in your home just in case. You may think you are against their use, but once you see how great they work in the hospital you might want them. Believe me when I say you won't want to stop on your way home from the hospital to get them.

Summary

Taking time to consider such serious issues as epidural use, bottle-feeding vs. breastfeeding, and who is going to take the day off from work when the baby gets sick is not the most fun way to spend a Saturday afternoon, but I implore you to take some time to do it. Many pregnant moms are apprehensive about discussing these issues and delay difficult conversations until they are in the delivery room or after the baby is born. Delaying the discussion simply adds to stress when the time for decision making comes. The fact is, like the baby, these issues are going to come out eventually. Ease the pain by thinking and talking *before* the baby arrives. Read on to discover more tips to get you ready through labor and delivery.

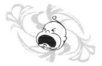

Chapter
Three

Uncensored Tips for Labor and Beyond

No matter how it happens for you — whether your water breaks at home and then the labor pains start, or you're induced or have a C-section — you may find yourself in need of a few inside tips. Here are some tips for your labor, delivery, and hospital stay that may make it all a bit more pleasant.

Listen to the Nurses

The first and most important tip is to listen to everything the nurses say. I say listen to the nurses because they are the people who will be with you for most of the time. They are also the people who have watched labor and delivery for years. They have a wealth of information; some know a lot more about labor and delivery than the doctors. Seek out their advice. And if they give you unsolicited advice, listen to that too. When they tell you how to push, pay attention. They know what they are talking about. The better you get at productive pushes, the easier your delivery will be.

Breathing Through the Pain

When I was in labor with my third child, I had a great nurse practitioner/midwife who was new with the practice. She was so supportive and helpful. She encouraged me to go with the labor and use my breathing. She wore a pin that said, "Listen to Women." She would say, "Listen to your body. You know your body, feel how your body is telling you what to do to have this baby." I felt very empowered. I can remember thinking, "I can do this, I can do this." Then I reached transition and I started to think, "I can't do this, I can't do this." I started to remember how the contractions come one on top of the other and how breathing hadn't helped one little bit during my previous births. It was time to call for Mr. Anesthesiologist, or as I like to remember him, "Superman."

Easy... I promise!

When you can't take the crying one more second, put the baby down in the crib. There's nothing wrong with taking a break. Our parents and grandparents considered crying to be exercise for a baby's lungs.

Superman

You must also know that it takes about twenty minutes for Superman to arrive at your hospital room so don't wait for the pain to become unbearable. Twenty minutes feels like twenty years when you're in pain. Ask for the anesthesiologist before the pain becomes overwhelming. You can always turn it down.

When my anesthesiologist came to the door during my third birth, I actually recognized him. He was present at the birth of my second child and he was good. My husband and I both breathed a sigh of relief at the sight of him. After he inserted the medicine he said that I would feel some "warmth in my bottom." I said to my husband, "I finally have a hot ass!" Relief came almost instantly. As Superman prepared to leave, I said, "Women must tell you they love you all the time." He said, "Yes, they do and quite often."

Easy... I promise!

How long before you can expect your baby to sleep through the night? It could be any time. Some babies as young as a few weeks old can do it. That's uncommon, but a few months is not.

Stool Softeners

After the delivery the nurse will likely give you some pain medication and a stool softener. Take them! "Stool softener?" you say, "Why would I need that?" Let me tell you: You'll probably find a bowel movement has never been so important to you before. You know when you are watching TLC and you hear the nurses telling the woman in labor to push into her bottom? Well, after a few hours of pushing into your bottom (and a tear or an episiotomy) that whole area is a bit "changed." That vaginal passage and the anus are a lot closer than you once believed, or wanted to even think about. The thought of passing a hard bowel movement through this very sensitive area will be enough to make you shudder! Not to mention the medical personnel who will all ask, "Did you have a bowel movement yet?"

Everyone gets so excited about it! They throw a party in the hospital for the first girl to have a bowel movement after giving birth. The stool softener really does help. Okay, I admit, they may not throw a party for you, but it will be one of your first steps toward feeling normal again.

Ice Pack Pads

After the delivery the nurse will give you ice pack pads (maxi pads that you crack and shake to make cold — voila!) for your perineum along with witch hazel pads and ointment to heal the site. Use them all! I would place the witch hazel pads over the ice pack and squirt the cream on top of the witch hazel pads. I would repeat this in the hospital as soon as the ice pack got warm. I also purchased a can of Dermoplast to bring home with me and I would spray the area with every trip to the bathroom. It was very soothing and promoted the healing of the site. Trust me when I say that the sooner the site heals, the better you will feel physically. The better you feel physically, the better you feel mentally.

Take the Products Home

Ask the nurses for more of any of the helpful products they give you so you can take them home. The nurses would wonder how I went through so many of ice packs so quickly. The truth is that I changed them as soon as they started to get warm because I found the cold so soothing. The nurses told me that the ice packs would only be good to use for the first twenty-four hours. That may be true, but the ice made me feel better and I used them even for the first two days at home. I brought so many home that even I didn't use all of them. I've actually used the extras as little ice packs for the kids when they get a bump or bruise. I just didn't tell them that it was a "Mommy maxi-pad ice pack." You can and should continue to use these products at home.

Pain Prescription

After the delivery, ask the nurse or doctor for a prescription for pain medication. The afterbirth pains can be alleviated considerably with it. You don't have to use them, but it is nice to know they are there. Of course, if you're breastfeeding, you'll have to bear the pain.

Start Recording

As soon as you reach the recovery room, start using your journal to record the times that your new baby eats, sleeps, poops or pees. Ask the nursery nurses if the baby drank any formula and write down when he ate and for how long. This notebook is also good to keep track of the gifts you'll be receiving. You may want to write thank-you notes. Gifts can be hard to keep track of once they start streaming in (and everything is harder to keep track of when you're sleep-deprived). You'll be able to easily write thank-you notes if you keep a record in your journal of who gave what.

The Nursery

It's okay to let the nursery take the baby so you can rest. Do not feel guilty, especially if you are not breastfeeding. Try to take advantage of the peace while you can; you will be up with the

Easy... I promise!

Pay close attention to the swaddling technique that the hospital nurses use. Ask them to demonstrate it for you. Being tightly swaddled is quite soothing to newborn babies.

baby soon enough. "Rooming in" is great as long as it is on your terms. Just keep in mind that this may be the only chance you are going to get to have some help in taking care of your baby through the night.

Women haven't always been left alone to care for a newborn. The novel *The Red Tent*, set in biblical times, discusses the tradition of all the women in the tribe gathering in the red tent to celebrate the miracle of birth. The women stay with the new mother for about a month and take care of the infant, bringing it to the mother for breastfeeding. The women pamper the

Easy... I promise!

If your growing baby is drinking a lot of formula or nursing for long stretches and still seems hungry, think about trying some rice cereal. If the baby's not ready, he'll just push it out of his mouth with his tongue.

mother so she can regain her strength and enjoy the birth of her child. I think a month of rest seems about right to start to feel healed up. What do we get today? As soon as the baby is born, the clock starts ticking; 48 hours (or even 24 in some states) and you're out of the hospital. When the time is up you will be sent on your way to care for yourself and your newborn along with the house, your husband, guests, and everything else you took care of before the birth of the baby. The red tent sounds good to me. I think a perfectly good tradition may have been left behind.

Nurse Instruction

Grab a nurse in private and ask whether she would be willing to explain to your family the list of duties you will not be able to perform for a while. Although you have just given birth, you and your family may still expect you to perform the same duties you always have. I asked a nurse to speak to my children on the day I was released from the hospital after having my third. She was happy to do it for me.

The nurses know the trauma your body has been through. They also have experienced going home after a birth or have someone close to them who has gone through it. Why not ask the nurse to talk to you, your husband, *and* your children about what mom will be able to do at home? My nurse explained to my older children that they could not expect Mommy to pick them up or do everything for them for a while. She further told them that Mommy needed her rest when she got home or she would be coming right back in the hospital. They don't give you this kind of tip when you do your Lamaze training.

Treat for the Nurses

On the day you are leaving the hospital have your husband pick up a treat for the delivery nurse and the postpartum nurse (a restaurant gift certificate, a box of chocolates, or a gift card). These people are often forgotten, but it won't be hard for you to remember how important they were to you at the time of your delivery and the first day of your recovery. Show them your appreciation. You may be coming back someday!

Don't Forget to Ask About Feeding

Ask the pediatrician the amount of formula that baby should be eating at this stage (for the next two weeks). You don't want to worry that the baby is not getting enough formula. At the two-week appointment you can ask again. If you're breastfeeding, ask how long you should breast-feed on each side. The nurses may send you home with some formula, which is nice. Those ready-made bottles are great, but outside the hospital they are pretty expensive. Ask the nurse for as much formula as you can get your hands on.

C-Section Hints

If you deliver via a C-section, here are a few tips just for you.

* Understand that the medications given during surgery will last for a little while and then wear off. Say "yes" to prescription medication that you can take in the hospital and at home. When you feel you can switch to ibuprofen, do it, as the other medications can be constipating.

* Although you will stay in the hospital for a few more days than a vaginal delivery you will still need to rest at home after a C-section. Stay away from the stairs, cooking, and cleaning. Consider looking into a postpartum doula.

* Clean your incision daily with soap and water. Keep a close eye on the incision, making sure there are no signs of infection.

* Make sure you have extra pillows on hand to help you sleep comfortably. The pillows will also help you to feed the baby more comfortably.

* You will still have some vaginal bleeding so be sure you are stocked up on maxi pads. Keep an eye on this bleeding, too.

* Try to move around a little bit each day. Movement will aid in the healing process.

* Insist you are treated with the same care given to any post-surgical patient!

Summary

Every woman's labor and delivery experience is unique. There are some parts of the experience, however, that are common to all of us. For example, knowing ahead of time that an epidural request might take a few minutes to be granted could be invaluable information for a new mom! Hopefully, these tips will help you to feel more prepared and make your experience more comfortable. I hope these ideas assist you in conquering the worst fear: fear of the unknown. Read on for a glimpse of those first few days at home with a newborn.

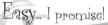

Easy... I promise!

Many women report a dramatic change in their relationship with their husband after the birth of their first child. Unfortunately, this change is not for the better. Give some thought to ways you can nurture your relationship with your husband after the baby comes home.

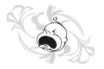

Chapter Four

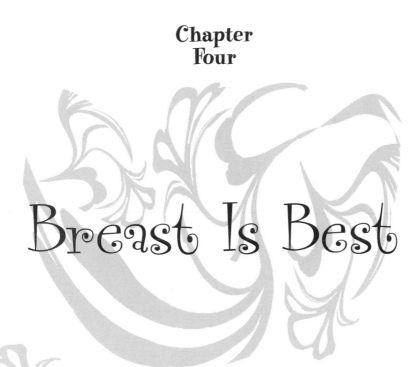

Breast Is Best

There may not be a more controversial issue for a new mom today than the big B. I am talking, of course, of breastfeeding. Everyone has an opinion on whether a new mom should breast-feed. The contributors are many: your doctor, your spouse, your friends, your mother-in-law, the guy who wheeled you into labor and delivery, the entire American Academy of Pediatrics and the most famous breastfeeding promoter of all, the nurse at the hospital affectionately known as "The Breast Nazi." When did your boobs become the object of worldwide opinion? One day your breasts are yours and the next they belong to your baby — and even, it seems, society at large.

"You just have to breast-feed the baby," everyone will chant. "There's no substitute for breast milk," you'll hear. It's like the *Seinfeld* episode where Jerry, Elaine, and the gang go out to the Hamptons to see their friend's new baby. "You have to see the BAAAby!"

They all repeat over and over. Similarly, "You've just got to BRRReast-feed!" It is what every new mom hears during her whole pregnancy. Other related mantras quickly follow. Among the most common mantras: "Breast is Best." "Breastfeeding is natural." "Breastfeeding is easy and convenient." Armed with such platitudes, moms go into labor confident of their breast-feeding abilities. Many think, "I'll give breastfeeding a try and see how it goes." What happens next may or may not be what a new mom imagined.

My lack of personal breastfeeding experience is why I compiled a little survey of friends, coworkers, and associates regarding their feelings and experiences on breastfeeding. Further extensive research was done online and offline. What I discovered is that the issues surrounding breastfeeding are many. The overwhelming pressure that today's mom feels to breast-feed, and the difference between breastfeeding myths and breast-feeding realities are critical concerns for many new moms. Of primary relevance is the variety of experiences. How can the same process be *soooo* varied from woman to woman? Finally, the interviews and research uncovered some terrific tips that will help a new mom who wishes to breast-feed successfully.

Oh, the Pressure

Today's mom does not really have a choice when it comes to breastfeeding. OK, maybe a mom has a theoretical choice. Bombarded with the tidal wave of sentiment, however, how many moms are able to say "no" to *the best nutrition there is on the face of the planet* the moment after their precious bundle is born? The answer is, not many. According to the U.S. Centers for Disease Control and Prevention, 77 percent of new mothers are breastfeeding their infants, the highest rate in 20 years.[1] The benefits of breastfeeding are publicized everywhere. Indeed, the publicity for breastfeeding is *so* effective that I bet that every man and woman could come up with at least three benefits of breastfeeding without breaking a sweat. I won't list all the benefits of breastfeeding here because if my theory above is true, you already know all the benefits! I will, however, mention that a new study reveals that breast-feeding can lead to a guarantee

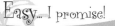

Easy... I promise!

"**Breastfeeding made me calm down and spend time with the baby.**"

that your baby will make millions, have a perfect body, and live to be 150! OK, I'm kidding, but just barely. Blogs, websites, newscasts, baby books, doctors, nurses, and every breastfeeding mom in existence sing breastfeeding's praises, insisting that every new mom do it! It's no wonder that many new mothers decide to go for it. The pressure can be a good thing. Breast-feeding *is* good. The problem can arise, however, when a new mom, armed with the simple mantra "Breastfeeding is natural" tries it for the first time and discovers that it is not as easy as she first thought.

In the results of my survey, 50 percent of moms said that, to their surprise, what they thought would come naturally did not. If 77 percent of new moms are breastfeeding their babies at birth, how many of those moms continue to breast-feed after they realize that breastfeeding is not as "natural" as they thought? According to a report by Brigham Young University in April 2008, only 36 percent of babies are breast-fed through six months.2 It seems then, that the pressure to breast-feed gets 77 percent of the moms started on breastfeeding, but the reality of breastfeeding for one reason or another keeps the moms from breastfeeding through the six months to a year that the American Academy of Pediatrics recommends.3 One way to make the breastfeeding experience a more successful one for women may be to take a look at some of the realities and myths of breast-feeding.

Easy... I promise!

"I was surprised breastfeeding did not come as natu-rally to me as it did for others."

The Breast – Feeding Myths

Myth #1: Breastfeeding Is Easy

The idea that breastfeeding is natural is absolutely true. The problem is that many women, me included, tend to equate nat-ural with "easy." The data say breastfeeding in the beginning is *not* easy. Although it may come more easily for some women (we like to call these women "SuperMoms"), the general con-sensus is that breastfeeding is a *learned* skill. Maybe pushing a baby out and expecting herself to immediately get her boobs to work to feed him is not the best strategy for a new mom to use when first breastfeeding.

Myth #2: Breastfeeding is Pain-Free

A further review of the data indicates that breastfeeding *in the beginning* is associated with some pain. Some of the pain report-ed can be severe. As Stephanie Wilder-Taylor notes in her book *Sippy Cups Are Not for Chardonnay*, "It hurts likes a rhesus monkey biting your nipples, only with more screeching — and not coming from the baby."[4] Well, then, there you have it: Breastfeeding can be painful in the beginning.

Myth #3: You Cannot Breast – Feed on a Schedule or Supplement

Easy... I promise!

> "I thought breastfeeding would be wonderful and I hated it so much."

One of the biggest myths about breastfeeding is that the breastfeeding can only be done one way. Not True. My survey of women breast-feeders tells me there are many ways to skin a cat when it comes to breastfeeding. Some women breast-feed exclusively the *attachment parenting* way.[5] Some breast-feed and pump so their baby can be given a bottle of breast milk while they are at work. Some breast-feed on a flexible schedule like the one described in the book *On Becoming Babywise*. Some women have trouble in the early weeks and give their baby a bottle, concerned that their breastfeeding days are over. With the right lactation specialist help, however, they are able to breast-feed for the next ten months. A practical strategy that includes a combination of help and useful information can be of positive value.

The Breastfeeding Truths

Truth #1: Breastfeeding is Convenient

One benefit on which women overwhelmingly agreed was that breastfeeding is convenient. The ability to be able to feed your baby at any time or any place with a free, perfect source of nourishment is truly one of breastfeeding's biggest pluses.

Truth #2: Breastfeeding Feels Good

Again, there is overwhelming agreement among the women who breast-feed that breastfeeding, once mastered, is "relaxing," "bonding," and "rewarding" just to name a few. Some have expressed the sentiment that they consider breastfeeding one of their "greatest accomplishments." One woman told me, "The ability to use my body to nourish my own child was just thrilling."

> Easy... I promise!
>
> "I found breast-feeding to be a unique, rewarding, and life-changing experience."

Truth #3: Breastfeeding Is Not for Everybody

Although there was a large percentage of women in my survey who did breast-feed and found breastfeeding rewarding, there was a smaller percentage who had quite the opposite reaction to their breastfeeding experience. Based on some of their breastfeeding answers, it was hard to believe that all the women were describing the same experience. These women told me that for them, breastfeeding was, "awkward," "friggin' painful," and "awful." Many of the women who had a negative experience felt much guilt, and that something was wrong with them. This makes me sad. It is a well-known fact that, for many reasons, some women cannot breast-feed. If you are one of those women or if you just don't want to do it, don't do it and don't worry about your decision. The important thing to remember is to feed your baby and take care of yourself.

Breastfeeding Tips and Suggestions

If the biggest myth of breastfeeding is that it is easy when it is not, it follows that the best way to successful breastfeeding is with education. Although many women read books before they go into the labor room, I think the overwhelming sentiment that breastfeeding is "natural" can lead a new mom to gloss over the material in *any* book. Based on my recent research, I am being told by breastfeeding moms that breastfeeding is absolutely *not* a natural and easy process but a learned skill. One way to learn the art is to watch another woman nurse. Grab a friend, family member, or neighbor who nurses and watch how she does it. Ask lots of questions. How better to learn how to do something than to watch a skilled person in action?

Easy... I promise!

"What surprised me most about breastfeeding was that I wasn't able to do it."

Another great idea to increase your success at breastfeeding is to find a lactation specialist or doula that your hospital or pediatrician recommends before the birth of the baby. (A lactation specialist may be covered by insurance.) Wouldn't it be great to see a familiar face to guide you in your first breastfeeding experience in the hospital? You've spent some time interviewing pediatricians whose philosophy you agree with, right? Why not take that same time to get to know a lactation specialist who you are in sync with, too. Take the time to find a specialist who understands your goals. You may be going back to work in six weeks; how can your strategy accommodate this need? You may want your husband to feed a bottle once a day; how can you keep your breast milk production up in order to accomplish this goal? You may want to feed on a schedule. You may want to breast-feed exclusively. All of these choices will affect the kind of lactation specialist you want to work with you. Wouldn't it be great to have a lactation specialist you know showing up after your baby is born to help through breastfeeding those first few months? Imagine the confidence you will have!

Summary

Breastfeeding is terrific. The choice to breast-feed is going to be the first of many decisions you will make as a new mom. If you want to give breastfeeding a shot, try not to get swept into all the pressure surrounding breastfeeding. Get informed by watching a nursing mom and asking lots of questions. Make the connection early with a lactation specialist who understands your personal situation and the place you think breastfeeding has in your life. Read what you can get your hands on regarding the mechanics of breastfeeding. Be informed. Know that breastfeeding is a learned skill, as well as a natural function that a woman's body performs. Most of all, remember, at the end of the day, your boobs may hold nature's perfect food, but they are still yours.

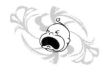

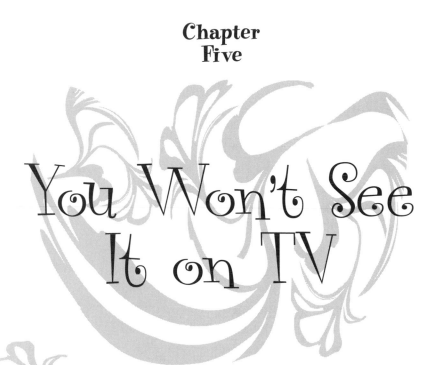

Chapter Five

You Won't See It on TV

Have you ever wondered why on TLC's *A Baby Story* the parents are never shown on the day they come home from the hospital? Why is that? What happens in those first few days at home with a new infant? It's not exciting, I'll tell you that. Each child is different, of course, but maybe this chapter will help you to find some commonality that will ease any fears of what is "normal."

After the birth of my third child, I recorded exactly what happens during those first few days. If I had to live through it, I figured someone could benefit from it. I had the presence of mind to record it because I had already started writing this book. One word of caution: There is a huge difference between how you feel when you bring your *first* baby home and how you feel when bring your *third* baby home. For that reason, I have included some flashbacks from the days after the birth of my first child, Joseph.

Those memories, as you will see, are still very clear in my mind.

Day One

My husband picked us up at the hospital with my two older children by his side. I had already asked the nurse to speak to my kids, and I watched as their eyes bugged out like saucers. After the nurse gave instructions to my older daughter and son about how Mom would feel, we started down the hallway. I was in a wheelchair carrying the baby and I remember the people in the hallway looking down and smiling at the happy family. We got to the car and I sat in the front with my husband as the baby slouched in the new infant car seat that was far too big for her newborn frame. I had piled folded receiving blankets in the bottom of the baby car seat to prop her up. She slouched. The new baby headrest was also in place. She still slouched.

Easy... I promise!

Use a journal to keep track of your baby's sleeping and feeding times. Record extended times of fussiness. The journal will help you to remember and think clearly when all the days and nights start to run together.

How times had changed. When we took the first Wolk child home, I sat in the back with the baby and held his sleeping head up the whole ride home. Baby three got no such treatment. I let her slouch while I rode in the front. This is what is known as third child syndrome.

We arrived home at about 1:00 p.m. We put the baby in her bassinet and I sat on the loveseat with my feet up. The neighbor children came over almost immediately along with their mother to see the new baby. This visit was fine because after the visit they took our kids with them to play next door.

We were in between homes and living in an apartment while a new home was being built. We were sick about bringing our new baby home to a tiny apartment but it turned out to have its advantages.

My husband and I put some frozen chicken and frozen vegetables in the oven for dinner. The baby slept most of the day and I woke her up at four-hour intervals to feed her. At this point the baby was eating three-quarters of an ounce to one ounce per feeding. I know this isn't exactly page-turning reading, but I said I would tell you the truth. This is the truth. How much your baby is eating is a very big deal, honest! Now I know why this stuff wasn't included in any of the other books I read. It's boring!

I felt good. I tried to be vigilant about keeping my incision clean and treated. I brought the squirt bottle home from the hospital and faithfully filled it with warm (not hot!) water to clean the perineal area. I felt ridiculous doing it, though, and hoped to God no one would come in and catch me in the act of squirting myself. The squirt bottle is one more thing no one tells you about.

I walked around gingerly and tried to rest with my feet up for most of the day. I felt that my emotions were steady. This was not the case, however, when my first child was born and I came home from the hospital.

Flashback: On the day I came home from the hospital with my first baby, I was pretty shaky. My parents came over that evening with cheese steaks (I'm a Philly girl!) to help us out. I barely got to the door to answer it before I broke out in tears. Just the sight of my father brought on this uncontrollable crying. He was not fazed, however. He looked at my husband and with me in his arms he said, "This is going to happen." My emotions were completely out of control. I think part of me wanted my parents to take me home with them instead of having to stay and take care of the baby. These uncontrollable tears subsided after the first couple days. After that I cried for real reasons like, "All my friends are out having a good time, and I'm stuck with this screaming kid!"

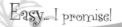

Easy... I promise!

The squirt bottle is your friend. Continue to use it at home after you use the bathroom.

As nighttime rolled around on our first night home with our third baby, I created a changing table (using a blanket) on the kitchen table. I would use this "changing table" in the middle of the night. The great thing about being in an apartment was that there were no stairs. Also, everything was a few feet from me. I could change the baby while the bottle was heating up.

That night, my husband brought the bassinet in our bedroom so he and I could sleep in the bed. After all, we had slept apart for two nights. I missed him. I offered to stay out in the family room with the baby, but my husband insisted we be together. We were just settling into bed at 11 p.m. when the baby woke up. I can remember actually exhaling with my husband's arm around me when the crying started.

She was up and kind of fussy but she had just eaten at 10 p.m. so I wasn't sure what to do. I took her out of the bassinet and we started walking around the family room. Some people call this "pacing the floors." Her crying did not wake my other children. I was relieved. I suspected while in the hospital that the baby might be cranky at night. At about ten the night before, she started to fuss and I said to the nurse, "Okay, you can take her to the nursery now."

This crying at night was the beginning of what ended up being a pattern for her. It's a common one. People describe this as the baby "having days and nights mixed up." I don't know if this phenomenon truly exists, but it sure makes sense to me. When you are pregnant, the baby is more active in your belly at night. During the day you rarely feel the baby kick because she is lulled to sleep by your activity. At night, on the other hand, you might even be kicked awake by these movements in your belly.

Easy... I promise!

After the birth, try to eat plenty of foods high in fiber. Plenty. That should make your experiences in the bathroom a bit easier.

After the baby is born, why should things all of a sudden change for her? This is the time she is awake, like it or not. Losing sleep was one of the hardest things for me to deal with. I was so busy during the day with my older children, caring for the baby, and the housework, that I would be my regular tired self around 10 p.m. I needed to change my strategy.

After the ten o'clock feeding, Ally seemed more awake than she had been all day, and, of course, fussy. I tried several rocking positions to keep her calm. Even though she had just been fed, she seemed to be uncomfortable. I checked her diaper. It was fine. I had just fed her so I was hesitant to feed her again. I made sure she was wrapped really tight in the famous "nursery receiving blanket wrap." I held her in the belly-to-belly position while I stood up and gently rocked her. I sat in the rocking chair and held her against my chest and gently rocked her. I also tried to lie on the couch with her against me while I gently rocked her. These methods would all work for a while and then she would cry again. She seemed to like the binky but even that would only work for so long.

After about an hour of changing positions I tried to feed her again, probably at about 11:30 p.m. This, of course, broke my cardinal rule (of feeding every three to four hours), but for newborns (and Ally was just

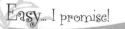

Easy... I promise!

Use your journal to keep track of the gifts people give to you and the baby. Someday you just might get around to writing thank-you notes.

about seven pounds) I find it is okay to try more food when all else has failed. In this case, she did seem hungry and ate about an ounce. I would try to put her down awake at stages during these two hours to see if she could fall back asleep on her own.

Day Two

At about 1 a.m., Ally fell back asleep. She was back up at about 3:30 a.m., not ideal but okay. I changed and fed her again. She fell asleep while I fed her and slept until about 6:30 a.m. I fed and changed her again and she fell asleep on the bottle again. I put her down and she slept until 9 a.m. I was feeling okay but tired. Each time I put Ally back to sleep, I used my squeeze bottle and changed my pad using all the creams and Tuck pads I could fit in my super-sized maxi pad — quite a sight! At one point I kept the Tucks pads in the refrigerator. They felt great — nice and cool!

On this day, a Sunday, my sisters-in-law came to visit, with a full course dinner in hand. They set everything up and cleaned everything up. They brought treats for the baby and for me. It's always nice to give a new mother something special, too. These are the right kind of baby visitors!

I pretty much rested all day while Ally slept, but I continued to wake her to feed her about every three to four hours. Joe's family entertained the kids and I kept my feet up while they all took turns holding Ally.

As evening came, I replaced the kitchen table with my changing table ensemble. I continued to treat Ally's umbilical cord with alcohol on a cotton swab. Don't be afraid to really get in there with the cotton ball, which leads to my next flashback. When Joseph was a baby I would dab the cotton ball just on the top of the cord. By the time I went to my six-week appointment, the doctor asked me to show him how I was treating the cord. It's never a good sign when a health professional asks you to demonstrate how you do something. Then he took a cotton ball and lifted the scab and wiped all the way around the base of the cord where it appeared red and raw. After changing my procedure and noticing no additional grimace on Joseph, I repeated this procedure and his cord came off 24 hours later.

On Day Two, Ally gave a repeat performance of the evening before, becoming fussy after the 10 p.m. feeding. We tried the same rocking and position changes as the night before. When the rocking did not help, I carried her around while rocking her. She fell asleep for good at about midnight. I gave her a bottle at 10 p.m. and one at 12 a.m. At each of those feedings, she only took about an ounce. I used to think that her fussiness actually made her hungry. Miraculously, when she woke at about 3 a.m., she fell right asleep on the bottle.

Day Three

On this next day, Monday, my nurse visited. She checked and

weighed Ally at about 10 a.m. I explained how much she was eating at each feeding. The nurse said that Ally was still slightly jaundiced and I should be feeding her every two hours. So much for my schedule! I asked if I should be concerned about the jaundice and I was told no, but that the more she eats the more she would flush through her system.

I adjusted my schedule to wake her to feed her every three hours during the day. Yes, I

> *Easy... I promise!*
>
> **Clean the base of your baby's umbilical cord with rubbing alcohol thoroughly each day. Don't be conservative. You want to dry it out so it will fall off.**

know this means that I did not listen to the nurse. During the day she still wanted to sleep right through feedings, but I woke her up. I know it may sound crazy that I woke a sleeping baby because "you never wake a sleeping baby," but I did it. I wanted to make sure she got as much food in her body as possible during the day and at regular intervals. It was my opinion that this process would help her to sleep longer at night.

My mom came to help on this day, a Monday. My son had to be driven to school and mercifully, a friend of mine who worked at the school offered to take him and bring him home for that first week. I didn't even have to ask. Casey had her first day of preschool (*Great timing, huh?*) and my mom drove me, Casey, and Ally to the preschool to witness her first school day. I was already feeling the pressure of having three kids and this made me realize all the more that doling out the attention to all three was going to be a challenge.

Casey also wanted me to do everything for her. When she

needed a bath and said, "I want Mommy to do it," my mom explained to Casey that she was going to bathe her. My mom told Casey that I was *her* baby and in order to take care of me she was going to do Casey's bathing and anything else that would make my life easier. I always remember that moment because I really needed to be taken care of and so often grandmothers side with the grandchildren and offer to take the baby. I wanted the baby! I also wanted my children to understand that I needed some help. They weren't the only one with needs!

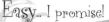

Easy... I promise!

Give the baby a sponge bath until the umbilical cord falls off and the circumcision heals. When you progress to bathing in an infant tub, be sure to test the water temperature with the inside of your wrist.

After Casey's bath, Mom kept Casey in the other room with her so that Ally and I could nap. Mom brought dinner with her and left in time for us to eat as a family. She returned the next day ready to do whatever was needed. She was at my disposal. She returned the day after that as well. This is the kind of help you need. It is *not* help if your company expects you to provide them with entertainment like some circus clown.

A Little Extra Sleep

Do whatever you can to get the sleep you need. I started to use little tricks to get some extra sleep when I could. I started getting ready for bed at 7:30 p.m. (at this point Ally was usually taking her evening nap). I would get into my pajamas, brush my teeth, and wash my face. I would also have Joseph and Casey in their pajamas and ready for bed. At 8 p.m, Joseph and Casey were put to bed for the night. Then I would get a blanket and my pillow and fall asleep on the couch until the baby woke up, usually around 9 p.m. or 10 p.m. This was hard to get used to since I would normally go to bed around ten or eleven, but the extra hour or two of sleep did seem to help.

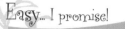

Easy... I promise!

Ask for help! All new moms need it. If a friend offers a meal or to take care of the baby while you take a nap, don't even think about turning it down.

During the evening my husband and I would dim the lights and lower our voices. Some have suggested turning the TV off when feeding at night so the baby will recognize the difference between nighttime and daytime. I tried that with our first child, but realized I was punishing myself instead of teaching the baby it was nighttime. Television was my new best friend. I started to look at the TV Guide for the week and see what would be on at two in the morning. "Ooh, *The Godfather* is on tonight!" I'd exclaim. Ever since then, movies have kept me company during baby time when the rest of the neighborhood and the rest of my family were sleeping. The trick is not to get so involved in a movie that you want to stay up and watch the rest of it after the baby has fallen back to sleep. I fell prey to that one night when the all-time chick movie *The Bridges of Madison County* was on. I was up long after Casey had fallen back to sleep because I had to find out whether Francesca decided to stay or to leave. At the time I can remember voting for the leaving. Get out, you fool, while you still can.

While Everyone Else Sleeps

Lack of sleep is an eye-opener, no pun intended! You start to think you're the only person in the world not sleeping. I can remember looking out our front window and cursing the dark windows of my neighbors, "They're all sleeping out there, the lucky bastards!" Don't worry, you'll sleep again too.

Summary

I hope this gives you some idea of what to expect. I may have overwhelmed you with too much detailed information, but it's all the details that can prove overwhelming in those first few days. Remember that each experience is different. The key is to be flexible and not to expect the baby to sleep through the night right away. Do not be surprised if the baby does sleep all day. Take care of yourself diligently. Demand the time you need to recuperate, and rest, rest, rest.

Easy... I promise!

Think twice before you bring your baby into bed with you. Babies get used to that treatment pretty quickly, and you could be creating a habit that you'll still be trying to break when your baby is a toddler.

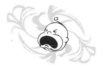

Chapter Six

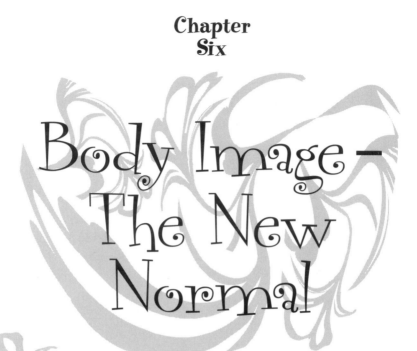

Body Image – The New Normal

For nine months, a pregnant woman watches her body go through this incredible transformation. There are a gazillion pregnancy books available that describe in amazing detail the physical changes in our breasts and our bellies throughout our pregnancy month to month. Where is the book showing our body changes for the months *after* we deliver? Once the little squirt comes out, no one seems to want to illustrate the putting of Humpty Dumpty back together again — please forgive the pun.

One illustration is clear, however, and that is that Mom is expected to put her figure back to pre-pregnancy shape but quick. I don't know where this unwritten rule was first born (I'm sure the guy who created bras and high-heels had something to do with it), but I think you will agree that getting back into shape after having a baby is as much a must for a new mother as is breastfeeding her baby.

As always, what society wishes us to do and what we actually do can be two very different things. Maybe in this case they should be different. A woman's body image after having a baby can affect so many other aspects of her life — her confidence level, her relationships, her feelings of normalcy, and on a practical level, her wardrobe. In addition to coping with her own body image, and what might now be possible and/or normal, a woman has to deal with the external pressure to lose weight.

Where does the pressure to lose the baby weight come from? Is achieving a pre-pregnancy shape even possible or is it an urban myth? What are some of the most successful ways a new mom can get back to pre-pregnancy shape? How can a new mom come to grips with her own body image? Some potential answers follow.

Those Darn Celebrities Can Do It, Why Can't I?

For some reason we expect our bodies to return to the exact same shape we had before we started the pregnancy process. Why do we have this expectation? Oh, I don't know. Could it be that we are bombarded with picture after picture of celebrity moms returning to pre-pregnancy shape in a matter of hours for their red-carpet walk at the Oscars? Could it be the plethora of books and magazine articles that scream at us every time we check out at the grocery store, the covers that insist that we exercise, stay fit, and be "hot mamas?" For example, did you see Angelina in her current pregnant state? She had not a trace of puffiness in her face or one extra layer of swelling on her ankles. Come on! Angelina as a representation of what the average mom should look like after giving birth? I think not. How can the average mother compete?

I believe we should forget about the celebrities. Cancel the subscriptions, stop watching the pre-Oscar shows, and most of all, turn off the E! channel. Torturing herself by staring at post-pregnancy images of Jen Garner, Nicole Richie, Gwen Stefani, J. Lo, Katie Holmes, and Christina Aguilera is absolutely no help to a new mom who is trying to put her body image into perspective. Who knows what these celebs are doing to lose the weight so quickly and who cares? The fact is that losing the weight is a priority for celebrities because of what they do for a living. Imagine the pressure they must feel and the lengths they are willing to go to look skinny after actually *being* pregnant. It is very upsetting to me that the media seems to reward the successful and chastise the poor souls who are not as fortunate. It is sad that these women are examined and picked apart at one of the most vulnerable times of their lives.

The issue here is not what the celebrities are doing to lose the weight, but rather the new standard their svelte pictures have created for the rest of us. Specifically, society and maybe (gasp!) our husbands may think and might even say (gasp again!), "Angelina can lose the weight right away; why can't you?" After removing your fist from your husband's gut after a comment like this, you might reply, "Once you start looking like Brad Pitt, you might expect me to start looking like Angelina." But I digress. All of the celebrity nonsense adds to the very real pressure women can feel to lose the "baby weight."

The Pressure to Lose Is Real

I believe the pressure to lose weight starts, ironically, while a woman is pregnant. I gained 50 pounds during my first pregnancy. It obviously took me nine months to get there. I make no excuses for this weight gain. I had never been so hungry in all my life. It was the kind of voracious hunger that comes with pain. I had to eat and eat I did. I had no issues while I was gaining the weight because, heck, I was pregnant!

At my six month appointment with my obstetrician, I started to feel the "weight pressure" for the first time. My husband and I went together to this appointment. I didn't even mind my husband being present for "the weigh-in." I had gained seven pounds in a month! *Yowza!* The nurse raised an eyebrow and said, "You had a big month this

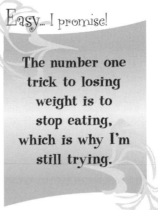

Easy... I promise!

The number one trick to losing weight is to stop eating, which is why I'm still trying.

month." I started to feel some sweat come on my brow. I kept my cool, though, and smiled big to my husband, not letting him know the fear that had crawled up my spine at the thought of my doctor noticing the weight gain figure on my chart and commenting on it. It's kind of like when you are in confession and you sneak a juicy sin in between two benign sins. I was hoping my doctor wouldn't notice the spike in my weight.

Once we got in the examination room and sat through the usual icing period, (where the doctor doesn't come right away but leaves you there to freeze in your paper gown while scraping at the files on the outside of your door making you *think* he is going to come in but he doesn't), the doctor knocked on the door and entered the room. He says hello to my husband and me and does his usual check of my belly, the baby's heartbeat, and my feet. *Please don't mention my weight, please don't mention my weight, please don't mention my weight,* I chant to myself, rhythmically wishing my appointment to come to an end. Just when I think I am in the clear, the doctor says, "Oh, I notice you had a big weight gain this month." My heart is now in my throat. *Please leave it at that, please leave it at that, please leave it at that.* The doctor goes on, "You really need to be watching what you eat. If you gain too much weight now it will be harder to lose later." When did losing the weight *later* become "Dr. High & Mighty's" concern?

As if I am not mortified enough, my sweet, sweet husband challenges the doctor on my behalf and says, "Doctor, she's only been eating the good stuff." (Keep in mind, with my husband's sweet tooth, he could have meant cake and ice cream.) Coldly, the doctor, who has packed up his little folder from hell, replies, "Then she is eating too much of the good stuff," and walks out of the room.

You know that dream you have when you are naked and you don't know it and everything is fine and dandy, and then you realize you are naked for the first time and you look at things completely differently? That's how I felt when the doctor made that insensitive comment. I felt completely naked and I knew it. I was going along happy in my pregnancy, not worrying about my weight and this ding-dong doctor pulled the rug out from under me.

The "weight pressure" is real. In her own way, every pregnant woman has felt weight pressure somewhere along her pregnancy: A sideways glance with a comment, "You really have four months to go? It looks like you could go tomorrow," or "You are *not really* eating for two, you know." And then after the birth, when you are just starting to feel not pregnant anymore, the dreaded, "When are you due?" The weight, no matter how you slice it, is an issue for pregnant and postpartum moms all over the world, and unless there is some huge rebellion against the magazine, television, movie, and entertainment rag industry replacing the beautiful people with the average people, the weight issue is here to stay.

The Truth Behind the Expectation

The truth is that every woman would like to return to her pre-pregnancy weight in as short amount of time as possible. Who doesn't want to look good, feel thin, and be in perfect shape? The truth is, it *is* possible to get back to your pre-pregnancy weight so don't let anyone tell

> Easy... I promise!
>
> **Losing weight is not as much a priority as it is getting into a routine.**

you different. As Stephanie Wilder-Taylor tells us in *Sippy Cups Are Not for Chardonnay*, "You don't need a book to take off the baby weight...losing weight after you have a baby is exactly like losing weight at other times."[1]

The best way to lose the weight is to take your time. In my personal survey of moms, almost 100 percent said losing weight was *not* their top priority. They were busy with other things like *learning how to be a mommy*. Losing weight according to these moms was, however, "on their minds." When you are ready, you can lose the weight. The trick is to take a minute — when you have a minute — to evaluate what *you* want. I needed to be ready. After a few weeks postpartum I started to get antsy for some movement so I put the chocolate down and I popped in a tape. I started moving. The movement felt good. I kept moving. Soon the pounds were melting away.

If losing the weight is important to you, set some goals of how you are going to get there. Keep in mind the American College of Obstetricians and Gynecologists recommends not even thinking about dieting for the first six weeks, especially if you are breast-feeding when you must consider establishing a good milk supply. They have, however, loosened some of the guidelines for the time that a mom can start to exercise. With a doctor's permission, they say, light exercise is fine as long as you feel good.[2]

Take the time to think about what you would like to achieve and how to do it. Do you need time alone to take a walk? Schedule some walking exercise into your week. Leave the baby with your husband or a friend or family member and stick to it. Do you prefer the gym for your workout? There may be babysitting services at local gyms that will watch infants, usually from six weeks old and up. Take advantage of your local YMCA to utilize this service. Do you want to stay with your baby while exercising? Invest in a Power stroller (you can even get these at secondhand stores), and walk with your little guy whenever you get the chance. Would you rather stay in the house? Forget about the dishes and pop a DVD in the player. Just moving around is going to make you feel good. Doing something for yourself is going to feel good. Studies have shown that exercise postpartum can increase energy and reduce depression, just like at any other time in your life.[3] The point here is to remember that if losing weight is a priority, you need to make it happen.

What If I Don't Want To Exercise?

It's possible that you are not ready to exercise. Knowing what you need to do (i.e., diet and exercise) and doing it can be very challenging. I don't know about you guys, but the second I would hear a little one waking from a nap, my arm would jut out to the bag of Dove chocolates I had at the ready, and I would pop chocolates like they were pieces of popcorn. Right after I started popping the Doves, I read that chocolate may not only add weight but also postpartum depression to my problems. Oops! I'm in the most vulnerable state in my life. I'm blue. I'm pudgy. I'm sore. I'm tired. And now I have to give up chocolate, too? I wasn't ready to give it up yet, so I didn't. The only thing I wanted to be told after having my baby was not to worry, that the weight will come off on its own. For many women, the weight *does* actually start to come off on its own. For one thing, you aren't so hungry anymore because there is not a baby in your belly. The relief of not having an insatiable appetite can do wonders for your figure. As well, it is a well-known fact that breastfeeding aids in taking off

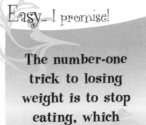

Easy... I promise!

The number-one trick to losing weight is to stop eating, which is why I'm still trying.

the weight. In my research, 85 percent of the women admitted that breastfeeding was the number one way they were able to lose weight. So if exercising is not on your agenda right now, I give you permission to put it on the backburner. You will get there in your own good time.

Summary

The pressure, both internal and external, for a new mom to "lose her baby weight" is pervasive and real, and for many new moms, upsetting. Moms need to take matters into their own hands and forget about comparing themselves to celebrity moms. Taking a minute to figure out what body image is important and what strategy is going to work for her is an important step. For some women, what is important is to leave the focus on weight loss on the backburner for now. That's OK. For some moms, getting back into shape as soon as possible is the priority. That's OK, too. Pregnancy weight can be lost. Luckily, breastfeeding alone will help the weight loss process along, as well as the fact that the hunger of pregnancy subsides soon after birth. Taking some time to get used to the enormity of the job of motherhood and being patient will also help the process along. The key is to define the "New Normal" for you and take the steps necessary to get there.

Chapter Seven

The Baby Commandments

There's nothing like a newborn to bring out the questions and comments from the peanut gallery. Everyone has something to say or ask. Here are a few of the more popular questions that friends, family, and total strangers may ask you:

* *Is she a good baby?* As if a baby has had the opportunity to be bad.

* *Are you getting any sleep?* Sure, these bags under my eyes are professionally installed!

* *Does the baby know night from day yet?* Absolutely, she just doesn't care about it.

* *Is your husband helping?* Well, he hasn't run away yet, does that count?

These are all relevant questions, but the most frequently asked question is this: How is the baby sleeping for you?

After I had a baby I understood why this question is so popular. Sleep — or, more accurately, the lack thereof — becomes the center of your universe. The important questions are the ones you ask yourself in moments of quiet desperation. When will the baby sleep through the night? What can I do to help the baby sleep through the night? How many hours of sleep did I get last night? It seems after two weeks of feeding the baby every two hours every mother has had enough, and rightly so. Who can function on just two hours of sleep at a time? Sleep becomes every new parent's obsession, and once you go through serious sleep deprivation you never forget it. That is why even strangers in grocery stores will ask whether you and the baby are getting any sleep. So when the hundredth person asks whether your baby sleeping through the night, remember that they got through it and so will you.

Easy... I promise!

An important note about husbands: The men on TLC do not actually exist. You know the ones. They coach their wives through labor and tell them how amazing and "heroic" they are. Weeks after the delivery they are calm, cool, and collected and look lovingly at their wife and new baby. If the guy who brought you home from the hospital behaves like a caged animal at every squeal your newborn makes, don't panic. This is normal. Lamaze is a required course, but "Babies Cry 101" is not. If all the crying is a shock to you, imagine how your husband feels.

How to "get" the baby to sleep through the night becomes one of the most valuable pieces of information that every new parent needs. If this information were sold on a shelf with a guarantee, it would make the inventor a mint. The truth is that there is no one answer to this question. In my opinion, there are many things you can do as a parent to aid your baby to sleep through the night as well as develop some other really good habits.

Sleeping and eating are two of the most essential functions your baby will perform for a while. They are also the *only* two functions they will perform for a while (unless you want to count peeing and pooping). What most books, friends, and doctors fail to mention, however, is that these important functions — how your baby feeds and sleeps from the beginning — can actually affect his ability to sleep through the night and develop good napping and eating patterns throughout his entire childhood. Understanding the connection between eating and sleeping patterns is the first key to surviving life with your newborn.

In order to help your baby develop good sleeping and eating habits, I have discovered a few fundamental rules. I call these basic rules the Six Baby Commandments because they need to be followed consistently from the time you bring your baby home. Keep these commandments and you can create a happy coexistence with your newborn that will last into the toddler years.

Now, take a deep breath, exhale, and prepare to accept these commandments in the depths of your soul.

* Thou shalt put the baby down drowsy (but awake) for bedtime and for naps during the day.
* Thou shalt give your baby naps during the day.
* Thou shalt wake the baby for "meals" during the day.
* Thou shalt hold the baby as much as you like during the day.

* Thou shalt burp your baby.
* Thou shalt not bring the baby into bed with you.

Commandment I

The first commandment is this: Thou shalt put the baby down drowsy (but awake) for bedtime and for naps during the day. This is a hard one, especially for new parents. It is a great temptation to wait until your baby is asleep in your arms before you put him down at bedtime or for a nap. Who is not familiar with the image of a perfectly peaceful baby sleeping on a parent's shoulder? However, you must remember, babies are going to learn what you teach them. If you teach your baby that she needs to be rocked and held close to your warm body to fall asleep, this is how she will learn to fall asleep. You will create a pattern of behavior that you will be enslaved to for an entire year, maybe even two. Frightened? You should be!

I fell headfirst into this "first child" mistake with my son. As a baby he required a whole sequence of events to fall asleep. First we bathed him, then we rocked him, then we rubbed his back in the crib, then we rubbed his back while holding him, then I lay on my bed with him on my chest and rubbed his back. Once asleep we would carefully place him ever so gently into his crib where he would instantly wake up crying at the feel of the cold sheets on his cheek. What kind of parents were we to place our sweet cherub's beautiful warm cheek against something so cold? We would immediately pick him up and start the whole process over. We started to try to figure out ways to warm the sheets so the temperature wouldn't be so different and startling. All of this from two CPAs! At one point all these steps did actually work, and it was taking us 45 minutes to get the kid to sleep. But then it stopped working.

Lesson learned! When our second child came home, I introduced her to the crib ("Casey, crib. Crib, Casey.") after she was about two weeks old. But from day one I put her down for bedtime and naps *in a drowsy state.* Not only did she sleep through the night at about eight weeks, but she never wanted to be brought near our bed. She would only sleep in her crib. We followed the same rule with our third child and she responded the same as our second child. Of course, there will be times when

> Easy... I promise!
>
> **It's okay to let your newborn sleep in his own room. Babies have a good way to let you know when you're needed – screaming and crying. You won't miss it, no matter how tired you are.**

your baby will fall asleep in your arms as you feed her. This is natural, especially with a newborn. When the opportunity presents itself, however, and a child is drowsy, don't wait to place her down until after she is asleep.

When your baby wakes during the night to be fed, you will probably change her diaper and then feed her. Your baby will probably fall asleep during the feeding and may even poop. Do you change the baby and risk waking her up? Or do you leave the baby and take your chances? It's a risk. If you leave the baby without changing her, she may wake up before normal time due to discomfort. This is often *not* the case. As Dr. Spock puts it, "A very few young babies seem uncomfortable when wet or soiled. Most don't mind at all."[1]

Along with putting the baby down drowsy at bedtime, there are a few corollary mini-commandments. After the early morning feeding (the one that happens around 5 or 6 a.m.), put that baby back to bed! I've met several mothers who would stay up with their baby after the 5 a.m. feeding. They felt that baby was having an "awake" time and was probably bored from sleeping so many hours straight through the night. Another mother I met felt that the baby was probably tired of being in the same crib and needed a change of scenery because she reasoned that she would certainly feel that way. "No, no, no!" I say. We can't compare how we would feel with how a baby feels.

Easy... I promise!

Why don't women talk openly about how they really feel about motherhood? Because they don't want anyone to think they're a bad mother.

Newborns need a lot of sleep. After the early morning feeding, put that baby back to sleep. I felt that 7 a.m. was a good morning wake time. Even if the baby woke up at 6:30 a.m., I would feed her and put her back to sleep until at least 7 a.m. This didn't always work, of course, and there would be days when we would be downstairs suffering through Barney at 6 a.m. with me on the couch and her in the bouncy seat. Eventually, though, she got the routine down and did not wake until seven.

The other corollary mini-commandment is, "Do not jump the first time you hear the baby stir in his crib." The greatest lesson you can teach your baby is how to get himself back to sleep. I espouse the "no monitor" rule. Trust me when I say you'll have no problem hearing the baby when he needs you. God provides him with his own monitor — it's called his wailing cries.

Commandment II

The second commandment is: Thou shalt give your baby naps during the day. Do not be misled into thinking that if you keep your baby up during the day she will sleep better at night. It seems logical, but it's simply *not true*! Well-rested babies sleep better at night. Babies sleep so much in the beginning because they *need* it. The average newborn is said to sleep 22 hours a day. Why do they need so much sleep? It is during sleep that babies do their growing.

Consult the following table for information on the relationship between the baby's age and the number of naps they need each day.

Nap Requirements by Age

Age	Number of Naps	Nap Length
4 months	3	4-6 hours
6 months	2	3-4 hours
9 months	2	2½-4 hours
12 months	1-2	2-3 hours
2 years	1	1-2 hours
3 years	1	1-1½ hours

Naps will become your lifeline. They are the only time you'll find during the day to nap yourself, pay the bills, clean the house, or even take a shower! Embrace naps, enforce them, and insist on them with your newborn.

Easy... I promise!

Your baby is going to learn what you teach him. By rocking your baby to sleep every night he is learning that he needs to be rocked to fall asleep!

Occasionally you'll run into a mother who says, "I don't know what it is, but my baby just doesn't seem to need naps during the day. She must not need a lot a sleep." Well, as my Nana would say, that's baloney. Any parent who says this is a parent who does not insist on the nap. Don't let that be you! For your sake and your baby's sake, insist on naps. If you're still thinking that you have *the* baby who just will not take a nap and doesn't need one, then ask yourself a few questions.

* Is the baby falling asleep too early in the evening?
* Is the baby waking up too early in the morning?
* Does the baby sleep through the night?
* Is the baby cranky during the day?

Answer these questions and then come talk to me.

A tired baby is a fussy wakeful baby. When it comes to babies, sleep begets sleep.

If you're putting the baby down for the nap drowsy but awake and he wakes up before a good nap, check on him and leave. All children can nap well; it's up to the parent to be the enforcer.

Commandment III

The third commandment is: Thou shalt hold your baby as much as you like during the day. I have read that babies who are held during the day gain a real sense of security and are actually able to sleep better at night because of it. Beware of naysayers. They will scare you with fears of spoiling your newborn. Such fears are completely unfounded during the first three months.

A 1995 study at the University of Connecticut looked at babies and mothers during the first six weeks and at one year. Researchers found that the babies who had more responsive mothers during those early weeks were more communicative at one year.

A study from Brown University in Rhode Island found that when mothers responded appropriately to their babies' cries during the first month, their children had higher language and cognitive scores at eighteen months. A 1995 study out of Manchester in the United Kingdom found that a rapid response to crying led to significantly less crying.[2]

The experts seem to agree: It is impossible to spoil a newborn up to a point. After about eight weeks — about the time the baby gets more comfortable in his own little body — his cries may be of a more demanding nature and less about his basic needs. In regard to spoiling, Dr. Spock has a bit of encouragement:

> Spoiling doesn't come from being good to a baby in a sensible way, and it doesn't come all of a sudden. Spoiling comes on gradually when parents are too afraid to use their common sense or when they really want to be slaves and encourage their babies to become slave drivers. Do not be afraid to respond to other desires of hers [the baby] as long as you don't become a slave to her. When she cries in the early weeks it's because she is uncomfortable for some reason or other — maybe its hunger or indigestion, or fatigue or tension.[3]

These studies tell us it's okay to trust your instincts to love and care for your child, to enjoy and embrace your child as much as you like. So hold your infant to your heart's content, just don't break commandment number one.

Commandment IV

The fourth commandment is: Thou shalt wake the baby to feed him during the day. I have found the amount of food a baby eats during the day affects the ability to sleep at night. They say a baby needs so many ounces per pound of his weight. You want the baby to eat at regular intervals so that he will get his recommended amount of food through the day and be able to sleep through the night. In order to do this you may have to wake the baby in the early weeks in order to feed him every three or four hours. Do it! The old adage says never wake a sleeping baby. I don't believe in the old adage, but I do have a new one to suggest: Never wake a sleeping baby *at night*. Wake the baby during the day to keep him eating every three to four hours.

Commandment V

Commandment Five is: Thou shalt burp your baby. That's right. Burp the baby — and often. Burp in between feedings. Don't put the baby down until after you get that burp. Burping can be done with the baby belly down on your lap, supporting his neck from the front and gently patting his back. Burping can also be done with the baby over your shoulder and gently patting his back. Sometimes the shift of position from shoulder to lap can force the burp. With my first I didn't realize how long it could take for the burp to come up. So I would give up and put him to bed. A little while later he would wake up crying with gas. After I realized what was happening I took time to get that burp. You can try burping in the middle of a feeding. This doesn't always work. You can burp whenever you hold the baby. I found it became a habit and part of holding the baby. Whenever I held the baby, I was patting his back.

Commandment VI

Commandment Six is: Thou shalt never bring your baby into bed. Never ever, ever, under any circumstances bring the baby into bed with you. If you teach her this trick you will never get her back in her own bed. I have friends who have bought cribs and beds that still have the plastic on them. They've never been used! If you start this trend you can kiss your sex life good-bye. Remember, you're not just preserving your love life for strictly pleasurable reasons; you may actually want to procreate again. This time, however, while your sweet cherub is living it up in your bed, you'll be in your closet trying to make cherub number two. Trust me, I speak from experience.

Easy... I promise!

To help prevent diaper rash, change your baby's diaper frequently. If a rash does develop, creams can be helpful – so can a little naked time. Exposing the diaper area to air for brief periods can help the healing process.

This is not easy for me to preach because I must admit to disobeying this commandment with my first child. He was just so darned cute. It seemed easier for him to sleep with us than to keep getting up to attend to his needs. It all started after his first birthday. I guess he was having some attachment issues at that point. In any case, we brought him into our "family bed." It seemed to work for a while, but then my husband and I noticed his jerky movements. Eventually, my husband would have to sleep face down (to protect the family jewels, lest they get kicked) and I would end up in the fetal position at the foot of the bed. My son needed lots of room to maneuver. One night, the last night of our rooming-in, my son kicked my face with such force that I ended up with a contusion on my eye. Don't let this happen to you. Keep the little ones in their cribs, safe and protected.

For all those naysayers who preach the "family bed" and its popularity in other cultures, I say, "We don't live in another culture."

Summary

One of the most interesting facts about the growth of a baby is that a baby's sleeping and eating habits are related. In other words, what and when the baby eats are related to how and when the baby sleeps. The Baby Commandments take this fact into consideration.

I: Thou shalt put the baby down drowsy (but awake) for bedtime and for naps during the day.

II: Thou shalt give your baby naps during the day.

III: Thou shalt hold your baby as much as you like during the day.

IV: Thou shalt wake the baby to feed him during the day.

V: Thou shalt burp your baby.

VI: Thou shalt never bring the baby into bed with you.

Carefully following these commandments is the first step in helping your baby sleep through the night and develop healthy eating habits. Remember, these are not mere suggestions. These are tried and true methods that work.

Chapter Eight

The Schedule

The direction to feed on demand is one that should live in infamy. It is the sole instruction provided by many pediatricians to moms taking home their new babies. Demand feeding sounds simple enough — baby cries, baby gets fed. To that, I say, "Baby poop!"

When I brought my firstborn home from the hospital, it seemed like he cried all the time. I had no idea what to do with him or why he was crying. I figured feeding on demand was the solution. I found I was constantly putting a bottle in the kid's mouth, but he was dutifully pushing it away with his tongue.

I wondered why my son was so fussy and not sleeping peacefully like I'd pictured him. Why was my child crying all the time and why wasn't the bottle fixing the problem? Why had I gotten pregnant in the first place? Would they take the baby back at the hospital if I asked them nicely? What did night and day mean anymore? It seemed all I did was feed the baby 24 hours a day. He was nothing like the content babies we saw in TV advertisements for baby food or baby soap or anything else.

My husband and I were near despair. If feeding on demand wasn't working, what would stop the crying? My husband and I agreed that the baby was not suffering from some "never stops crying disease," so we called the doctor and he suggested changing formulas. "Maybe his stomach can't handle the iron," he said. We were told to give the new formula 48 hours before we could look for a change. "Forty-eight hours!" we exclaimed. "That is a lifetime." After the 48 hours, our newborn was screaming as heartily as ever. "Change the formula again," the pediatrician said. "Maybe the baby can't handle the lactose." Are you kidding me? All of these years of medical school and all they have for me is, "Try changing the formula?"

I was sinking and sinking fast. We wondered why the hospital didn't give us a baby manual on the way out. We sure needed one. When we expressed our frustration, we were told, "All babies are different." *No (baby) shit, Sherlock*, we thought. We knew all babies are different but we figured there had to be some basic guidelines to follow.

After more than enough crying I thought maybe I was the only one who left the hospital with Damien and all the other babies were perfect, happy angels.

Finally I spoke to my mom and cried through my quandary. She had recently spoken with a girlfriend whose daughter had the same problem with her baby. She gave my mom a schedule — the same one she'd given her own daughter. It was a baby schedule her pediatrician had given to her 35 years earlier. It had worked for all six of her babies and for her daughter's children. I couldn't believe that in this, the Information Age, I had to go back to the 60's for something typewritten on an old Corona to find salvation!

The schedule turned out to be the single most useful parenting tool I ever received. It could be used for breastfeeding or bottle-feeding mothers. I don't exaggerate when I say it saved my life.

Here was a plan I could follow — one that every pediatrician seemed afraid to give out for fear of arrest by the lactation police. The fact is, I wanted someone to tell me what to do. Some of those less creative women, like me, really needed strong guidelines to follow. Rules, regulations — what else could a red-blooded American accountant ask for? My response to the schedule was "Hallelujah! No more guess work."

The schedule outlined a feeding schedule for the baby month by month. For the bottle-feeding mom, it identified the number of ounces the baby should get. For breastfeeding mothers, it specified how long to breast-feed. It identified how long the baby would sleep and how long the baby would be awake during the day, month by month. It suggested the introduction of foods at the appropriate months. I had entered Nirvana.

I believe the schedule is *the* reason my son and my two daughters slept through the night from 10 p.m. until 6 a.m. at eight or nine weeks. Basically, the schedule says to feed the newborn baby every four hours at the given times of 6 a.m., 10 a.m., 2 p.m., 6 p.m., 10 p.m., and 2 a.m. It is my theory that over the first eight weeks of life the baby's "clock" is getting adjusted to night and day. Once their little bodies adjust to the "clock," they've got it; they can sleep through the night. So the question is, do they have enough food to keep them satiated through the night? By feeding them throughout the day at regular intervals they will be eating the proper amount so that by eight or nine weeks they will weigh enough (ten to twelve pounds) and their bellies will hold enough to skip the 2 a.m. feeding.

It's true, but most doctors will never explain this. Apparently they prefer the baby be up for the first year of her life at her whim. Whatever the baby demands, they say. Why put the baby on a schedule when she will tell you when she's hungry?

The problem is babies cry for many reasons and not all their cries are hunger cries. Crying is their way of exercising, of telling

Easy... I promise!

Mothers can be critical of one another. If you heat your baby's bottle up in the microwave, make sure you shake it well, and make sure you don't tell anyone you do it!

you when something is in their diaper, of just plain something to do. How is a brand new mother supposed to know when a cry from her baby is a hunger cry? Sometimes the baby will cry because she is uncomfortable, tired, wet, *and* hungry. You can't assume the cry is a hunger cry — especially if it comes just an hour after you've fed her.

I assumed all cries were hunger cries, and I was feeding my son constantly. He never got a good feeding at one time, so he was probably not getting enough food over a 24 hour period. In addition, he wasn't sleeping at regular intervals and was cranky and gassy from all the food I was forcing on him.

Once I started to use the baby schedule as a *guide* things fell into place. My son was taking a good feeding at each feeding. I tried to hold him to eating every four hours, but if he truly seemed hungry (and now I could start to tell the difference in his cries), I would feed him at three hours. I would put him down at regular intervals to nap but would wake him at the four-hour mark (at the latest) to feed him during the day. At times, I could follow the schedule to the letter and at times I couldn't. I discovered that was okay.

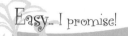

Easy... I promise!

Remember: Always put the baby down drowsy but awake for naps and night- time sleep.

The schedule is a basic guideline. If the baby wakes in the morning at five instead of six, feed her. See if you can steer her back to eat at 9 a.m. instead of 8 a.m. to get a little closer to the 10 a.m. mark. Keep feeding at regular three-hour or four-hour intervals — whatever seems to work for you and your baby. Make sure you are putting the baby down *drowsy* to nap at regular intervals during the day and make your last bottle around 10 p.m.

It takes some work, but the results are amazing! After approximately eight or nine weeks your baby will be sleeping at mostly the same time every night and feeding at mostly the same time every day. There will be fluctuations of course, especially if the baby gets sick. Just roll with it and use your common sense and steer her back on her schedule.

Now schedules, as you already know, have gotten a pretty bad rap over the past few years. It seems as if no doctor, lactation specialist, or even the writers of the humorous books on childcare dare to espouse a schedule. I suspect this is because it is politically incorrect to tell people what to do, especially where their children are concerned. Perhaps they're afraid that if we put all children on the same schedule, we will usurp their individuality.

After doing some research on the subject, I found that the

creation of the schedule in the 40s was actually a response to serious intestinal infections that affected tens of thousands of babies a year. Doctors felt that the babies were getting sick due to a combination of contaminated formula and irregularity in feeding so they suggested putting the babies on a regular feeding schedule. The pasteurization of milk took care of infections. Parents, however, were so traumatized at the possibility of their babies getting sick that they continued feeding on a strict schedule. Both parents and babies were miserable. As so often happens in matters such as these, the tides turned in the completely opposite direction away from the schedule and stayed there. The era of demand feeding was born.

Part of the swing away from schedules is an attempt to put the control of mothering back where it belongs — from the doctor to the mother. Schedules were shunned to prevent doctors from exerting control in an area where they did not belong.

The ironic thing is that the demand-feeding rule (which I thought meant feeding the baby every time he cried) actually came from an experiment performed in the 40s that proved feeding schedules were quite natural. In the experiment, doctors wanted to see what kind of a feeding pattern a baby would develop if left to his own devices. What was discovered was that a baby after about the first two weeks will develop a more or less regular "schedule of feeding" and a reasonable one at that, approximately every three to four hours.[1]

Why are the critics so afraid of schedules when they turn around and insist that parents provide a schedule in adolescence to provide youngsters with a secure environment? If a schedule is good for the adolescent, then it is good for baby. I suppose it has to do with keeping the process natural. Even other mothers share this flawed advice. "Accept the first few months of sleeplessness as inevitable and give your baby a chance to find her natural rhythms."[2] I submit that a feeding schedule is the most natural thing in the world. Everything in nature is on a schedule. We ovulate on a schedule, we experience pregnancy on a schedule, and heck, even labor is on a schedule.

Even Dr. Spock talks about the "misunderstanding about the relationship between self-demand feeding and schedules." He goes on to explain: "The main purpose of any schedule is to do right by the baby and another purpose is to enable the parents to care for their child in a way that will conserve their strengths and spirits."[3] Conserve their strengths and spirits? I like the sound of that! Thank you, Dr. Spock, for confirming that. Parents don't have to discount their needs completely when they have a child. Any of my mom's friends could have told you the same thing, but to hear it from Dr. Spock gives the idea added weight! I shared the idea with my husband and I took it to heart. Life became a lot easier.

Another good reason to develop a schedule is so you can get out. The sooner you have a solid schedule to follow, the easier it will be for other caregivers to watch your baby. It will actually be a pleasure for them because they have detailed instructions of what to expect. This is especially helpful when you have older children and you *have* to leave the baby. I know that at first you can never imagine leaving your baby so why worry about someone else having to follow a fly-by-night schedule, right? Wrong!

> *Easy...* I promise!
>
> **After the birth is a good time to watch some funny movies. While your hormones are going crazy and you're feeling sad for "no reason," a few laughs will give you a little pick-me-up.**

Even if you're not going back to work, you never know when you may be needed for an emergency or an event that you just don't want to miss. Consider your possible caregivers — your relatives. If they know that at six months your baby still does not sleep through the night, takes an hour each night to rock to sleep, rarely takes naps, and sometimes sleeps in your bed with you and your husband, they're not going to be too interested in helping out when you need them. Watch all your relatives fly to the hills when they catch word that you need a sitter for an extended period of time. You won't be able to find anyone willing to go through the hoops you're willing to jump through to care for your baby.

Keep this in mind before you dismiss the notion of a baby schedule. The sooner you have a solid schedule to follow, the easier it will be for other caregivers to watch your baby. Your family members will be thrilled when you can leave instructions on what they can expect from your baby, including feeding times and sleeping times. They will enjoy their first experience so much that they won't pretend they are not home the next time you need a sitter.

I know that there are skeptics out there. "All babies are different," they will say, "How can one schedule work for all babies?" Believe me when I tell you the schedule can work for all children, no matter their temperament, or whether they are breast- or bottle-fed. I have friends who have bottle-fed (as I did) and friends who have breast-fed, and all were able to use the schedule successfully. One of the most popular features of the schedule is that by using it you eliminate the need for "crying it out" — a solution to getting your baby to sleep through the night that many "experts" require after your baby is about six months old. My babies never had to "cry it out;" they slept through the night in the earlier months and continued to do so because of the schedule.

Some parents really take the schedule to heart. They find out how well it works and after witnessing its success, they ostracize themselves and their babies from all social functions and get-togethers with friends and family — from everything and anything that interferes with The Schedule. I have heard of people leaving family gatherings abruptly before dinner is even served to get Suzie in bed to stay on schedule. Others leave Mass before it's over, or they abandon full carts of groceries in the grocery store. They will even leave a line right before they reach Santa to preserve the sanctity of The Schedule.

Even if you're not that rigid (and you don't need to be!), do not be surprised if your adherence to the schedule annoys some people. After all, you are not the first people to have a child. Why do you get to leave early? "But the schedule," you'll protest. "The schedule demands respect." Yes, the schedule demands respect, I agree. However, the beauty of the schedule is that once you've established the schedule, it stays in place, even if you vary it from time to time. It's okay if a nap is missed or shortened once the baby's clock is set (eight or nine weeks) because she's still going to go to bed at about the same time and sleep through. You will not destroy the schedule once it has been established. Please do not ostracize your family and friends. You can have a life and have the schedule, too.

Summary

Putting my son on the schedule was the best thing for both of us. He became very secure in his regular feeding times, his naps kept him from being cranky when he was awake, and I got my life back. I could do things around his schedule and actually get the things done. I didn't have to spend all night for months deciding whether or not to feed him a bottle because after nine weeks he didn't get up for one. The point is that the feeding, napping, awake time, and sleeping through the night are all connected. No one told me this. I was in the dark in the beginning and that made me feel panicky. *Is it going to be this way forever?* I wondered. *Will he be awake around the clock and I'll still be guessing what his needs are?* With the schedule, things started to fall into place.

A new baby sends everything into a bit of an uproar, but over time, the schedule will help bring calm to the storm. I assure you that my babies are not the exception. The schedule will work for your baby, too.

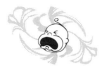

Chapter Nine

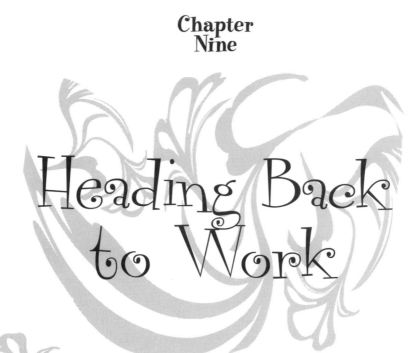

Heading Back to Work

If having a baby is hard, going back to work after having a baby is even harder. For many new moms, there is no option, it is back to work they go. Other mothers are happy to go back to work after their six weeks at home are up. If they are like me, when they returned to work, they left skid marks in the driveway. Regardless of a new mom's reasons for returning to work, the actual return to work is a whole new world. Remember in the movie *Working Girl* when Melanie Griffith finally got the job she wanted and she's lounging in her swivel office chair with the music, *Let the River Run*, by Carly Simon playing in the background? I wonder how she would look if she had left a baby behind that morning. Again, if she was like me, she probably kept swiveling and maybe even jumped up and down a bit, but I digress.

After a baby, things have changed for the working girl. She is no longer on her or her company's timetable; she is on her caregiver's timetable. Where once she could focus only on her work, she now may be distracted by the care her little guy is getting, that runny nose she noticed while dropping him off, or that breast-milk that is dribbling down the front of her blouse. Is it possible to smooth out some of the rough edges for the return to work? You bet! Included here are some ideas for making the transition back to work a little easier. A discussion of how to handle the workload as well as how to handle changes in coworkers is included. Finally, tips on letting go of the pervasive guilt that new moms encounter are presented.

Letting Go of the Guilt

If you are a new mom returning or planning to return to the workforce, you are not alone. In a recent U.S. Census Bureau report, 55 percent of new moms were part of the labor force.[1] Clearly, returning to work soon after a baby is a reality for millions of women. The guilt that comes with leaving a baby is also a reality. There are the moms who *must* work and feel guilty for leaving their little ones. There are the moms who don't feel guilty for leaving their little ones to continue in their career, but they feel guilty for *not* feeling guilty. Although I joked earlier about "leaving skid marks" in the driveway on my first day back to work, the truth is that I *did* feel guilty. I was one of those moms who felt all through my pregnancy that I was going to return to work, fit my baby into my working life, and continue on my way to "having it all."

I was delusional. Once the baby came, leaving him wasn't as easy as I thought it was going to be. Oh, I'll admit that at first I did enjoy being able to enjoy a cup of coffee in peace. After the novelty of my private cup of coffee wore off and the reality of leaving my little guy day after day sunk in, I was very upset. In short, I felt guilty.

After a few weeks of torturing myself I realized something. The guilt was getting me nowhere. My son was in good hands. My neighbor, a mother of five, was watching him in her home every day. The fact was that I *needed* to work and there was nothing I could do about the fact that I needed to work. Feeling guilty about a situation that I

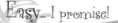

Easy... I promise!

I have felt guilty everyday since I returned to work for some reason or another.

had no power to change put another weight on my shoulders and sapped my energy. It was unproductive. The same can be said for the guilt of women who *want* to work. They cannot change the fact that they want to continue working. Working for them is who they are and affects the kind of mother they are. Leaving a job for the sake of a child when the result will be a miserable mother is not an answer. The guilt, again, is unproductive.

When I started to realize the negative effects of the guilt, I changed course. I started to focus on the things I *could* change to make my working life a little bit easier. I started to try to enjoy the time I *did* have to spend with my little guy. The guilt started to recede. No matter what your reasons for returning to work, put the guilt on a shelf and leave it there. Focus on the things you *can* do to make your working life a bit easier when you return to work. Luckily, there is good news in the way of help for the working mom.

Company Help

Never before has corporate America been so accommodating to the working mom. According to a *Redbook* article, "two-thirds of big U.S. companies have some sort of family-friendly option."[2] You've heard the rumors of flexible schedules, on site day care, and lactation rooms, haven't you? Well, here's rule number one. Take advantage of *everything* that is offered by your company. It is popular for companies to exhibit their family-friendliness. Learn what goodies are offered by yours. Although I realize that every new mom does not work for a Fortune 500 company, the climate no matter what the company is generally family-friendly. So, even if there is not a formal list of family friendly options, you may be surprised to find that goodies may be offered if you simply ask. Remember, corporations do these things because they need good, experienced, and hard-working employees. If providing these benefits satisfies that need, they will not only enthusiastically market these goodies to the employment pool but also expand and improve them.

The first goody I would like you to find out about is a flexible schedule. Some companies offer more than six weeks or twelve weeks leave. Some also offer a flexible schedule after twelve weeks at their discretion. The additional leave probably will not come with pay, but it may include benefits. See what you can work out. It is my belief, as long as your finances allow, that the longer you can have a flexible schedule for the first year of your baby's life the better. When we first become mothers we tend to think of the care of our babies in terms of *forever*. Instead, focus on reaching the six month mark and then the year mark. For the first six months you may have the baby with a family member or an at-home nanny. This kind of situation may be the best situation for a newborn. After six months, however, as your little guy grows, a daycare close to work may be a better fit for your family. Having a flexible work situation for those first six months to a year can help your peace of mind and in turn your performance on the job versus working a full-time schedule during this stressful time.

In order to capture the flexible job situation you have to be proactive. Come up with a schedule that can fit your needs as well as your employer's needs. Call for a meeting and sit down with your boss for a chat. While I was pregnant with my son, I hadn't broached the subject of my maternity leave with my boss. As I approached my third trimester, I realized I needed to have "the talk" with him. I called a meeting and sat down across from his desk. I simply said, "How would you feel about me coming back to work for half days after my six weeks are up for a full five months?" He looked at me and breathed a huge sigh of relief. He thought I was going to tell him that I wouldn't be returning to work at all after I had the baby. He agreed to my plan.

Easy... I promise!

Ask. You never know what they may be willing to do to accommodate a good employee.

The point here is to ask! In my case, although my pay was halved, I was able to keep my job and my benefits. My son was six months old by the time I returned to work full-time. Working full-time with a baby on a schedule and sleeping through the night is a much easier proposition.

Family Help

Everyone *says* they want to help with a new baby. They'll say, "Just let me know what I can do and I'll be here for you," or "If you need me just call." Yeah, yeah. You never ask for the help and they never come. Suddenly you are left wondering why you are sitting among five loads of laundry, a dirty kitchen, and a bathroom that should be condemned. This is not the time to be shy. Get specific. Ask lots of people little things they can do to help. "Mom, can you commit to watching little Tyler on Mondays from 7:00-5:30?" instead of "Mom can you babysit Tyler until he turns eighteen." Or "Dad, can you commit to bringing Tyler home on Tuesdays so I can get to the gym and work off the baby weight?" How about, "Sis, could you drop by on Thursday nights to help me fold laundry while watching *Grey's Anatomy*?" Believe me, if they can't do it, they will tell you. Move on to the next person on your list. Remember, the help that you request doesn't have to be forever, just until you get your groove back.

Easy... I promise!

"There was tearing going back, but I was passionate about my work."

Overwhelmingly, working mothers have told me that the biggest help to their returning to the workforce was the help they had from spouses, family, friends, and neighbors. The different scenarios and creativity these gals have used to "make it work" are astounding. Some women worked at night and had their husband watch the baby so they could work. Some had their parents and in-laws watch the baby for a few months before putting the baby into daycare. Some paid an in-house nanny to be in their home so the baby wouldn't have to be taken from the house. Some paid their cousins to clean their house to lighten the load of housework. The key to all of these examples is that each of these women asked for the very specific help they needed.

Tips While on the Job

Once you are back at your job on a more or less regular basis, you may find that things have changed a bit. While you are still the go-getter you always were, you may be panicking as five o'clock rolls around because you still have two hours worth of work and you have to leave to pick up your little guy. Your coworkers may be a little jealous of the fact that you are leaving more or less on time — never mind the fact that you came in early, worked through lunch, and did not engage in one "non-work" conversation. You may feel slighted because you missed a meeting at eight o'clock at night. Welcome to the Working Mom World.

While I'd like to tell you that your career is going to be on the same path that it was before you had a baby, I would probably be lying. Unless you have a full-time nanny at home, chances are, your career track may have to slow down a bit. In corporate America, the workers who can stay late and travel at the drop of a hat are the ones who keep moving ahead at a frenetic pace. That's no reason to throw in the towel on your career though. Remember, your little guy is growing a bit more every day. The increased need for you to be home at a reasonable time will not be forever. In the meantime, I've put together a list of tips from personal interviews to help you get through these next few months on the job unscathed. I believe these tips can be useful in any work situations.

* ***Try not to be late.*** You want to portray the image that all is well and everything is under control to get your boss, peers, and or staff comfortable with your reliability.

* ***Communicate.*** Keep good communication with your staff, project team members, clients, and most especially, your boss. Publish your availability. Make sure everyone you have to deal with has your phone num-

ber, email, and schedule so if they need to reach you they can. Do not give anyone a reason to question your schedule or say, "We don't know where she is today."

Easy... I promise!

Any mom who has had her daycare lady pry a crying baby off her as she walks away in tears knows it's no way to start your day.

* *Keep the status of your projects updated.* Letting your boss know the status of the projects you are working on will give him or her the confidence that you are making the transition back to work successfully. As BabyCenter tells us, keeping in touch with your boss this way, "not only keeps you boss informed, but it's a useful way to keep a record of how much work you accomplish from one week to the next."[3]

* *Stay organized.* To be successful in any job requires organization at home and at work. My college roommate tells me a working mom has to be one step ahead. She suggests having two black pants at the ready in case you get puked on and have to change two minutes before you leave in the morning. She also suggests keeping your gas tank filled at all times. It causes extra stress when you know you are running late and have to fill up. She jokes that she can live five days in her minivan if she has to.

* *Establish a baby schedule.* As described in Chapter Eight, a flexible baby schedule can be a life-saver for a working mom. The possibility that your baby could be sleeping a seven-hour stretch by 9 to 12 weeks is a big advantage for the working mom.

* *Beware of the tattletale.* Every company has a tattletale. The one person who spies on you and catches you at the exact moment you walk in the door five minutes late. This is the person who is just turning the corner cubicle to catch you as you are trying to sneak out at 4:45. In the 80's movie *9 to 5* starring Lily Tomlin, the tattletale was a woman named Roz. Whenever the girls in the office wanted to talk about their boss, they would head to the ladies room and talk, but not before they checked under the stall for Roz's feet. The tattletale does not care that you are trying to juggle a new baby and a demanding career. She spends her days ferreting out those who do not conform so she can tell her boss, ostensibly to make herself look better.

I had a tattletale when I started back to work. I can't even remember her name. She was a miserable older woman who was friendly to my face but was charting my every move. My boss at the time was managing from a satellite office and was only in my office about once a month. Anytime I punched in at 8:05, he was on the phone with me about it. I couldn't figure out how he did it until one day I called him on it. "How can you know when I am getting in the office?" I challenged him, "You are in Dallas." "Oh," he said, "My spies are many." I found out later from my own office connection that it was the job of our office tattletale to call him every morning with a report of who came in late.

The best way to handle the tattletale is to give her nothing to tattle about. Do whatever you have to get in on time. Attend all meetings with your head held high; no frazzled stories of how you almost didn't make it out of the house. Keep everyone on your staff informed of your schedule. Above all get your work done without shifting your workload to everyone else. In most cases, those you work with are not as concerned about your new mother role as you are. They want things to be "business as usual." If it is at all possible, keep it "business as usual." Be the same professional you were before the little person arrived. Your professionalism is what made you successful in the first place. Most of all, remember to take good care of the next woman on your staff who becomes a mom!

Get your sleep. Sleep is critical at this stage in your life. Hopefully, your baby is on a schedule and sleeping through the night. This does not mean that you can use the time while he is sleeping to do extra work. Do not fall into the trap of so many working mothers. In trying to do it all, they come home from a full day working, take care of their family, wait for the family to sleep, and then work into the wee hours just to do it all over again the next day. Sleep deprivation is dangerous. I'll say it again, *Sleep deprivation is dangerous.* In addition to the obvious dangers such as falling asleep at the wheel of a car from exhaustion, there are many other dangers. Lack of sleep can lead to hypertension, weight gain, heart disease, and even death. Sleep deprivation is used as a form of torture for goodness sake! It affects one's cognitive ability, which certainly can not be a good thing for one's career or family. So, please, do not use those late night hours to "catch up." Your sleep is *not* negotiable. If you find that you need those late night hours to "break even," I insist you re-evaluate your situation. Pay a sitter so you can stay at work later and finish your work there. Cut back on your workload until things calm down a bit. Hire a cleaning person so the bulk of the house cleaning is done. Do anything you have to do to get your sleep. You are far too important to your family to risk your health.

Summary

If you are a working mom, you are not alone. Whether you can't wait to get back to your post or you are going back to work kicking and screaming, the good news is that there is help for you to take advantage of. Ask your employer what kinds of flexible schedule they might offer you for the first six months to a year of your baby's life. When you do head back full-time, remember to get your sleep. Try to stay as organized as possible and keep the lines of communication open with your staff, your clients, and your boss. Keep good track of your workload and try not to bring it home. Arrange for an after-hours sitter one night a week and stay late if you need to get work done during the week. Stay flexible. The situation you need at this moment may not be the situation you need forever. If you need more time off right now, ask for it. Pick up the additional hours when you can. Most of all, leave the guilt on a shelf. Guilt is useless. Enjoying the time you have to spend with your baby is priceless.

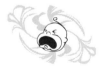

Chapter Ten

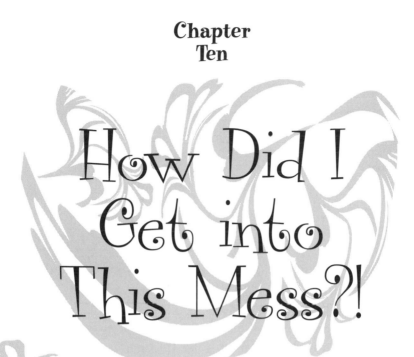

How Did I Get into This Mess?!

When you bring your first baby home from the hospital and start to experience what the job entails, it can be, well, a bit frightening. Surreal thoughts may creep into your head. I wonder if the hospital will take the baby back? Exactly how many years do I have to do this? There is no question that you love your child, all mothers do. It's just that you may not have realized the enormity of motherhood. Even if you have a lot of experience with other people's children, it is different when it's *your* child. Only your own baby will have you cursing your sleeping neighbors or sleeping husband in the middle of the night as you pace the floors. This chapter will examine the feelings you might experience as motherhood begins and some ideas to make the transition easier.

When I was 12, I didn't think that taking care of a baby was such a big deal. My best girlfriend and I used to babysit for the neighbor who lived down the street. The mom stayed home. The dad was a construction worker. They could probably just barely afford the modest split-level house they bought. Once a year they went out to dinner to celebrate their anniversary, and I vividly remember one of our experiences babysitting for them. This particular time, their two older boys (ages five and three) were not a problem, but the third, a baby, was another story.

> **Easy... I promise!**
>
> The show *Supernanny* is a great source of parenting advice and ideas. If you haven't heard about "the naughty chair," it's time to tune in.

He cried the entire time. I don't remember being upset about it. I just remember thinking that maybe something was wrong. We contacted a higher authority: my girlfriend's mom.

When she arrived she didn't do much more than we did to calm the baby down. She simply held him and walked around the house with him in her arms, commenting on the squalor of each room she walked into. (I still remember there was a plate full of Oreo halves in the kitchen. Yes, it is exactly what you are thinking. Someone had "teeth-scraped" the creamy middle out of the Oreos and left the cookie halves for later. Waste not, want not, I guess!) My girlfriend and I had of course noticed the general disarray but didn't think much of it. Oh, how the adolescent mind works!

My friend's mom eventually left us to rock the baby, and we waited for the young couple to come back from their big date. We never thought to call the mother knowing that this was probably the only time this year she was going to get out. This was my first real peek into the world of the housewife/mother.

I didn't give it much thought. My girlfriend and I took our money and thought about how to spend it. After all, we didn't have to deal with the situation day to day. We could walk away.

It's one thing to visit a place. It's quite another to live there! Fast-forward 13 years. I have a child of my own, a son. I took no time off before the birth, and I actually went into labor while at work. Two days later, I came home from the hospital with my newborn and I looked around for his mother. I was immediately thrown into the world of babies, housework, and housewifery. One of the easiest ways I can sum up the change that all new moms experience is that you can no longer go to bed when you want to. Instantly you are on some one else's timetable.

No one can prepare you for the changes in lifestyle that you'll experience when that first child is born. I remember wondering whether I was supposed to be undergoing an instant metamorphosis into this new person named "mom." It seemed like it should happen the moment a child is born, but it wasn't that way for me. I didn't feel like a mother, and I wondered when my own transformation would begin. I wondered if a beam of light would come through the ceiling like in *Close Encounters*.

It wasn't long before I began worrying that I was a bad mother. All of those feelings I'd heard women on TV talk about saying they are instantly bonded the moment they gave birth did *not* describe what I was feeling. Sure, he was cute and all, but I was feeling other emotions a little more strongly — like anxiety, nervousness, and panic. I kind of felt like there was this new sea outstretched before me and I wasn't quite sure if I was going to like it, how I was going to handle it, or even how to begin to stay afloat.

To go from complete freedom to complete responsibility for

another human being is unfathomable. I started to marvel at my parents. How had they been able to do it? Why would anyone want to do this? I also wondered whether my husband was going to continue coming home from work or whether he would opt to escape. That seemed logical to me. This demanding little person cried almost constantly when he wasn't sleeping. I began to think all of the television shows I'd seen about the joy of babies were full of soup (my grandmother's polite way of saying "full of shit").

> Easy... I promise!
>
> **Don't neglect to do nice things for yourself after the baby is born. Take a bath. Get a pedicure. Have coffee with a friend. Make it happen. Don't wait for someone else to suggest it.**

Perhaps your "before baby" experience is like mine. I used to get up in the morning, prepare myself a cup of coffee, shower, do my long hair (condition, mousse, dry, and curl), drive to work, work a full day, come home, and put my feet up. After my first was born, I was lucky if I got the shower. I was 25 and stuck in my brand new Colonial house with my hot red Acura gathering dust in the driveway.

Maybe I am too young to start having children, I thought. There has actually been some discussion of whether the raising of children is harder on younger mothers or older ones. I don't buy it. I was relatively young and I had a very hard time adjusting. I used to think that maybe if I had waited until I was a little older I would be more relaxed, better able to cope. Apparently this isn't true either. The truth is that you go through it when you go through it, and your stress is the same whether you experience it now or later.

For a long time I wondered why motherhood is so hard. My aunt used to say that God makes it that way to ground you — to keep you home for a while with the baby and to force you to bond. Let's face it, if the baby were pleasant and happy on its own all the time, we would be off taking care of our own needs just like before the baby was born. Maybe my aunt is right. Maybe the baby requires so much attention in the beginning to bond you to the child. You have to give of yourself completely and put your life on a shelf for a while and say, "Bye, bye life, see you later." Whether that's the reason or not, I know you may frequently ask yourself this question: How am I going to do this for the next 18 years?

Millions of women out there experience feelings of distress in their new role. It's not that you don't love the little bundle; it's that you are insecure in your ability to care for him. What if I can't wake up every night when I am needed? Or the more immediate issue may be, what if I can't get off the couch?

On the bright side, aren't we better prepared than ever for motherhood? Women of our generation are in the unique position of entering the world of mothering with the cocky opinion that we've got it all worked out. We were brought up to establish our careers and own our homes and go on vacations with our husbands *before* children. This was our mother's dream for us. We've experienced some success in the hardnosed workplace. How hard can taking care of one child be? Add to this confidence the plethora of information available on the subject of childcare and pregnancy through books and the Internet, and we expect instant success.

Our mothers went into this pregnancy and childcare thing without the benefit of our generation's new bible: *What to Expect When You're Expecting*. We have no hang-ups about going back to work after the baby is born. There are plenty of good daycare facilities out there. Things will be the same as they always have been, just more complete now that our baby has arrived. Right? Wrong!

Of course, it's not that easy. It never has been easy, and it never will be easy. Our experience may be a little different from our mothers' experiences, but it is not easier. Some difficulties no longer exist, but new ones replace them. Oh well. The good news is that there is help. Some of the best ideas are the ones that have been around the longest, even with all the books and websites out there. Pick and choose at will.

It would be great if new moms would ask for the help they need, but most won't. Every mother I know feels she should

Easy... I promise!

Your journal is good for more than just baby stats. Keep track of your feelings. Get your thoughts on paper. If the thoughts feel scary and too private to ever reveal, you can always write them down and then burn the piece of paper. Sometimes just writing it down is cathartic.

be able to handle motherhood alone. You're just out of the hospital, you're sore, and you've just got to get up and take care of the baby. You're not the first woman to have a child, you think, and all the other women who have gone before you seem to handle it without a problem, so you will, too. You need the new mom mantras.

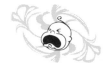

New Mom Mantras
Mantra #1: Manage Your Visitors

Although your very first thought when you get home from the hospital may be to climb into bed with your newborn, not so fast. Your first challenge may be how to handle the baby visitors. Naturally, everyone will want to come and see the baby. Most mothers would agree there are two kinds of baby visitors. Type one is the baby visitor who wants to see you and the baby and bring a gift. (Hopefully, there will be some gifts that are just for you. I call these gifts "treats.") The type two visitor is the visitor who has come for an afternoon outing and wants to be entertained. Embrace number one, shun number two!

Everyone is going to want to come and visit. Visits are fine as long as they are on your terms. This is your new family we are talking about. It's okay to say no to your relatives who may want to visit the day you come home from the hospital or immediately thereafter. You and your husband and your baby are in new territory. Take the time to establish the ground rules for your precious new family.

My advice is to pack 'em in at the hospital. At the hospital, there are specific visiting hours and you can't entertain because you'll be in bed. It may also be a good idea to mention your wishes before the baby is born.

You may feel some guilt over this decision. When feelings of guilt creep in remember that you've just had a major procedure that required hospitalization. Speak up. Why at this particular moment in your life do you have to worry about everyone else's feelings? Think about yourself and your baby.

Of course, every rule has exceptions. You may feel up to company the minute you return from the hospital. After I had my first child, I remember my roommate in the hospital leaving before her 48 hours were up because she missed being home. Can you imagine? Leave the constant help of the nurses who swaddled my beautiful baby boy with the utmost precision, took him to the nursery so I could sleep, and brought me glorious menus from which I could order breakfast, lunch, and dinner all prepared by someone else? No way! After 48 hours,

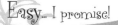

Kids thrive on routine. Be as consistent as possible.

they had to carry me out of my hospital room, my fingernails gripping the doorframe and scratching the walls as they carried me down the hallway. If you do desire company in your home after the birth of the baby, then I say go for it — just be certain it is on your terms and you can recline like the Queen of Sheba. Okay, so you make it through the visitors and then something even worse happens — they all leave you alone. It's your first time alone all day with the new joy of your life. Your husband goes back to work for the full day. All the relatives are on to their daily life and you are left alone to chart your own course in your new role as mother. Maybe you will go back to work in six weeks or maybe you won't. The fact remains that at some point you will experience the first day of your new job. Like any new job it is accompanied with a certain amount of anxiety. Unlike other new jobs you cannot leave it at 5:00 p.m. or even 6:00, 7:00, or 8:00 p.m.

Mantra #2: Take It Slow

I know you are used to taking on a million things and actually getting them done. The only thing you have to do now is take care of yourself and your baby. You're recovering from a procedure that required hospitalization. You are not expected to clean the house, do laundry, and cook as soon as you get home. Take these days to rest and to get to know your baby. Hopefully, you are writing down feeding and sleeping times and following the Six Baby Commandments. Taking a shower will be the big accomplishment for the day. Congratulate yourself if you can get this done and try not to worry about the dust gathering around you. Oops, now I've done it. I reminded you about the dust.

If you and your husband have already bought your dream house, you may now have a problem. Our generation seems to take an inordinate amount of time keeping our brand new homes in pristine shape. The house always seems to need to be in model condition because this is the way we were first exposed to our house. We walked through a carefully staged model home and so we try to duplicate the effort by spending hours at the local accessory stores buying stuff to re-create that "model-home" look. This look is difficult to keep up day by day.

After a baby, that kind of upkeep is impossible. Those days are gone. Old habits die hard, however, and you'll be tempted to keep up the model-home look by cleaning at every chance you get, specifically while the baby is sleeping. While you used to have endless hours to clean on the weekends, you now have little bits and pieces of time to do the same amount of work.

> **Easy... I promise!**
>
> Take a shower when you can. You might find it easiest to jump in the shower before your husband leaves for work. If that doesn't work, there's nothing wrong with letting the baby cry in the crib while you take a quick shower.

Frustration will quickly set in if your husband, who knows you've been home all day, innocently comments with the most common question that new fathers ask: What did you do all day?

Hold fast. Your job is to take care of the baby and yourself during the day. Once the weekend rolls around, your husband will start to get the picture about how much actual energy the little one takes. Capitalize on this knowledge and communicate again with your spouse. Explain to him that your job during the day is to take care of the baby and his job during the day is to go to his job. When he comes home you can both take care of the baby and whatever else that you can do *together*. If the baby is safe and taken care of at the end of the day, you have done your job.

Realistically though, you will find an uncontrollable urge to do some cleaning and laundry. Take it slow. By following the schedule you will start to figure out the times of day the baby naps. You can use this time to pick and choose the chores that get done. For the first few weeks, though, the baby might not be in any kind of schedule so free time will be rare. Try not to get frustrated. Remind yourself that if the baby is safe and cared for, you have done your job for the day.

When you absolutely have to get something done, do the basics. Empty the dishwasher, do a load of laundry, wipe down the toilet seat. Don't think of chores as something you will need an hour to accomplish. Break them up into steps. The most important areas of your house are the kitchen, the bathrooms, and the laundry room. If you keep these areas in reasonable shape you're in good shape. Let the dust sit. Dust never hurt anybody.

Mantra #3: Never Pass Up a Nap

Never pass up a nap. Naps will become very important to you at this time in your life. You are getting less sleep at night — and it is *broken* sleep. Naps will be your lifeline. If you can't nap, then rest with your feet up. It really does help. Naps will become your husband's lifeline, too. How, you ask? Well, if you nap during the day, you'll have energy for sex at night. I wanted to start a new movement when I was home with my children. I called it "nap for sex."

It seems new mothers are passing up sex because they are so tired by the time evening rolls around. Dr. Laura Schlessinger in her book, *The Proper Care and Feeding of Husbands,* says that "by turning their husbands down for sex, women are passing up their own orgasms."[1] Hey, I enjoy an orgasm as much as the next person, but the tiredness new mothers feel is real! It's not just that we're tired and don't want pleasure; it is just that the work it takes to get there is often outweighed by the pressing demands of our family. You may feel like many women do. If your husband did more around the house, then you wouldn't be so tired and might have energy to have sex. But that idea holds no water, either. The truth is that even if the husband did do more work around the house, the woman would simply move onto more projects that need to be addressed. The result is the same. The woman is still tired, and the man is getting no sex. My solution is take a nap.

I know: Napping is a rather taboo subject. It's almost as big a secret as masturbation. No one admits to taking naps. Why be ashamed? Everyone does it! You should enjoy your naps. Embrace your naps.

I needed a nap up until the time my youngest turned three. That represents ten years of naps. Most women wonder when I had time to nap. I would nap when the baby napped. I followed the schedule so that the baby would nap in the morning and in the afternoon. During the afternoon nap I would usually lay down. Most women would spend this precious time to clean. But really, what would your husband like more — a clean house or more sex? Sadly, some women might say a clean house. For those women I offer my condolences. Other women might say he expects both. To those women I would say, he may expect both but he ain't gonna get it for a while, so he needs to choose. You can choose for him. The answer is nap, nap, nap. Dr. Laura would be proud.

Easy... I promise!

Make date nights with your husband, even if you can't go out because you're unwilling to leave your newborn. Make dinner together or rent a movie you've been dying to see (preferably something exciting so you'll stay awake). Just remember to be flexible. If a fussy baby interrupts you, don't hesitate to try again another night.

Mantra #4: This Too Shall Pass

After two weeks of your new life, you may be starting to feel it. The original euphoria may be wearing off and you may be thinking about the next eighteen years with some regret. The baby could be showing her true colors, and as she's adjusting to her new surroundings she's getting louder and more demanding. The sleep deprivation is kicking in and maybe a little depression. You may feel lonely and overwhelmed.

It is time to remember that this too shall pass. Chant it to yourself if necessary. When these feelings start to creep in, tell yourself that you will get through this. Let's look at a few tips to help you through the transition. First, follow the baby commandments and the schedule. You will probably not be able to follow the schedule to the letter. Stay with it. There will be good days and bad days. If you try to follow the schedule consistently, you will see results.

Call a friend or family member just to talk. I called my mother every morning after my daughter was born to report her sleeping progress. My mother would respond with encouragement. It was helpful to have someone to talk to about it. Stay connected to the outside world.

Easy... I promise!

Keep the judgment to a minimum. Watch out if you find yourself saying, "I'll never act like that mom." You don't know what you'll do until you're in that situation. Who knows? That could be you bribing your kids with candy in the checkout line.

Even if it means a two-second phone call to a friend or a walk around the block where you hook up with a neighbor, it will help. Do what you can to feel more plugged in to the outside world.

After the first few weeks, sleep may become a major issue. The urge to do it all on your own might be passing as you wonder whether you'll ever get sleep again. It might be time to speak to your husband about taking shifts. If you are bottle-feeding, try calling it a night at 8:00 p.m. Let your husband take the 10:00 p.m. feeding while you sleep until the 2:00 a.m. feeding. My husband and I tried this with all three of our children and it worked out great. The advantage is that you get a lot more sleep. The disadvantage is that you lose the early evening together and falling asleep together. If you feel the disadvantages of this idea are too great, then just try this solution a couple times a week when you feel you need a boost.

If breastfeeding, see if your husband will wake up when the baby wakes up, change the baby, and then bring the baby to you to breast-feed. After the breastfeeding your husband can bring the baby back to her crib. Okay, stop laughing. These are just ideas. I have a girlfriend whose husband actually did do this.

Mantra #5: Ask for Help

After a few sleepless months you may not mind sharing your bundle of joy with the outside world. One great tip is to ask a relative to stay overnight one night with you. The relative can stay up with the baby in another room of the house and take care of the baby's needs for one night. One night of uninterrupted sleep is a precious gift. If you are breastfeeding, maybe you could use this time to supplement through the night with a bottle to get that full night's sleep. (Be careful that your milk supply is well-established before you try this.) Maybe the biggest help to you would be to have someone help clean the house or provide you with a dinner. Granted it's tough to ask for such things, but if someone close to you sincerely offers help, take them up on it. You can always return the favor.

Why?

Sometimes it helps to remind yourself why you decided to have children in the first place. Why do people have children? How do they go about making this decision? Of course, I asked people. For any woman over 55, the answer was simple: "We didn't decide. I just got pregnant." The absence of birth control will do that to a woman. Since the advent of the Pill, however, it seems that people make a conscious decision whether or not to procreate.

How do people come to the conclusion that they are in fact "ready?" I asked around. Some of the answers were interesting:

* "I wanted to share my life with a child."
* "I wanted to experience having a child."
* "I wanted to express my love for my husband by having a child."
* "I was feeling incomplete."
* "I wanted to have family and all that entails."
* "A child loves you unconditionally."
* "When a child wakes up, the first person he wants to see is you."
* "They smile at the sight of you."
* "They run to you when they see you."
* "They look for you throughout the house."
* "The sound of your child laughing is the most wonderful sound in the world; you'll do anything, say anything to get that child to laugh."

I wonder how many people would actually have children if they knew what it was going to mean for their own lives. In the end, after all the guesswork, the answer became clear to me. I was in the car with my husband and three children. We had just finished breakfast at a restaurant, and my youngest said her big brother's name clear as a bell for the first time. My husband and I looked at each other, like we've done a million times before when the children have said or done something sweet or humorous, and smiled. A warmth washed over me and I realized that this is the reason we have children — to add this meaning, this dimension to our lives that we would never have in any other way. Children are what life's all about!

This doesn't stop us from gritting our teeth a thousand times a day at the many frustrations raising another human being can bring. Unfortunately, this grinding of the teeth usually brings guilt. That voice inside your head starts spouting off the same proverb that those strange older women in the grocery line can't help but share with you. You know, those older women you don't even know who come approach you in stores when you are with your children

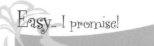

Easy... I promise!

If you don't have any close friends who are moms, consider joining a local moms group.

and share their unsolicited advice. "Enjoy this time with them, it goes so fast." That's what they say, and that's what the guilty voice inside your head may say as you grind your teeth.

But your question likely remains, how can I enjoy this time when I'm so damn frustrated all the time? I must not be a good mother. Why is it so hard? Dr. Spock says this:

> Of course parents don't have children because they want to be martyrs, or at least they shouldn't. They have them because they love children and want some of their very own. They also love children because they remember being loved so much by their parents in their own childhood. Taking care of children, seeing them grow and develop into fine people give most parents — despite the hard work — their greatest satisfaction in life. This is creation. This is our visible mortality. Pride in other worldly accomplishments is usually weak in comparison.[2]

When your baby finally smiles at about four weeks, you get it. You'll do anything to get that smile. It *is* all worth it. Okay, it's mostly worth it. How can one smile from this mostly cranky human being bring so much joy and pleasure? This is one of God's miracles, no doubt. I'm convinced God gives us that smile to keep us in the game.

Summary

I hope this chapter has given you a frame of reference for how you may be feeling as the reality of motherhood first starts sinking in. Remember first and foremost that you are not alone. All new mothers have feelings they don't want to have. The feelings that you are having are normal and have been felt by all the other mothers out there at one time or another, even if they don't admit it.

> If you don't enjoy staying home, you're not alone. Many women choose to stay home because they feel like that choice is best for their families – but they don't all love it.

Many women have written their honest feelings on this subject in their books. Check them out in my resources section if you get a chance. If you are looking for more immediate input, there are scores of mom message boards on the Internet where new moms are talking to each other live every day. Read through some and find one that matches your personality and feelings on motherhood. There are also message boards that are community-based so you may actually be able to hook up with other new mothers in your area. My favorite message boards are listed in the resources section as well.

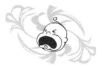

Chapter Eleven

What Is a Housewife and How Did I Become One?

Webster's Ninth New Collegiate Dictionary defines *housewife* this way: "1. a married woman in charge of a household; 2. a small container for small articles." I'm not making this stuff up!

You may not realize it when you get pregnant, but you become more than a mom after giving birth. The transformation that takes place is more sinister then Dr. David Banner's transformation into the Incredible Hulk. As soon as you set foot in your home with a newborn, you will be faced with the reality of a life-altering role change. In one fell swoop you are no longer an independent working woman; you are now, dare I say it, a housewife!

What was once a word used to describe those "other" women that you would see in the mall pushing their children in strollers and standing in line during your lunch hour, is now a word defining *you* — housewife! In a little while you may begin to think about your relationship with this label, a label whose connotation may be unclear.

Whether you'll be home after the birth of a baby for six weeks, six months, or six years, you will have to deal with the "housewife" label. Never does the line between roles seem as clear as it does when your husband walks through the door asking, "What's for dinner?" Your response may be to look around and wonder whether he's speaking to you.

How did you get to this point? It's a question we all end up asking ourselves. What is a housewife and how did I become one? In my opinion, the housewife role and the expectations the name implies is as much a

Easy... I promise!

Give your baby white cloth diapers to snuggle with as they sleep. The cloth diapers grow softer with each washing, and a replacement will always be available if one gets lost or misplaced. Bleach them and it won't look like your child is walking around with a filthy rag as they grow older.

part of the transition in becoming a mother as dealing with diaper rash. Unlike diaper rash, however, there is no cream available to smooth away the "rash" that is sometimes caused by the job of being a housewife. (That makes me think of *The Full Monty* and one of my favorite movie lines: "Anti-wrinkle cream there may be; anti-fat-bastard cream there is not.")

The question became quite real to me when my son was two years old. My personal life was at odds with my professional life. I could no longer stay late at work, and sometimes I had to excuse myself from meetings. I was clocking in after the 8:00

a.m. start time, and I generally felt that I was not doing either job in my life (work or mother) well. So I did what many of my Information Age sisters did: I cashed out my 401(k) and vacation pay, put my suits and heels in the closet, and joined the stay-at-home mom world.

Let me tell you, *I was scared*!

The transition was not a smooth one for me or for my spouse. Unfortunately for my husband, the first episode of *Oprah* that I watched was about a divorce case. More than just a divorce case, it became a kind of "indictment"[1] of the stay-at-home mom. Is she or is she not a true full partner in the marriage? In the case discussed on *Oprah*, the "corporate" wife sued her successful husband for divorce and requested half of their millions.

I wondered how the producers could make a whole Oprah episode out of this case. But I watched on and learned that getting half of the family's wealth was not a slam-dunk for the at-home mom. After I picked my jaw off the floor, I marveled as the studio audience, women no less, expressed their view that the at-home mom's work was an "honor and a privilege." Ouch! And that the money belonged to the husband because he had in fact "earned" it. Double ouch!

I was astonished. I wondered whether I had just magically been transported to 1950. But there was more. The lawyers in the case expressed the view that the wife could not have earned the same amount of money as her husband on her own. Further, they said she was entitled to what her husband was willing to give her. At this point I looked like the character Ted Striker in the movie *Airplane*, when he learns that he has to fly the plane alone. (That is, sweat is literally pouring down my face.)

I couldn't believe my ears. I thought, *Who is to say how much money she could have earned? She could have been the next Madame Curie, right?*

When my husband came home that night he found me crouched in the corner of the foyer ready to pounce on him like Spiderman. I wanted to know how he felt about this issue: Did *he* feel this way? Could I picture him in a courtroom with a bunch of suits saying that he "didn't think of our marriage as a team effort"[2] as the successful millionaire husband had said? Should I run back to my old office to get my job back? After I calmed down, he assured me of two things. Number one: We were blocking out the channel that provides *Oprah*. Number two: He did not feel the same way as the lawyers in that divorce case or as the members of Oprah's studio audience. After a few hours of soothing, I resisted the urge to call my boss and get my old job back. I stayed out of the full-time workforce and I'm glad I did.

The way women feel about leaving a job behind — even temporarily — and the impact that staying at home has on a marriage is at the heart of adjusting to the role of motherhood, yet few people discuss it. Remember the *Brady Bunch* episode when Bobby Brady started to think Jesse James was a hero because all the violent parts of the Jesse James movies were edited out? (I think almost any real-life situation can be related to a *Brady Bunch* episode.) Well, mothers need the whole picture without any editing. Making a successful adjustment from working woman to mother is vital, yet most of the books on motherhood tend to leave out this discussion. These books delve into the discussion of adjusting to motherhood only when they talk about postpartum depression. Well, what about all the rest of us who are not suffering from postpartum depression but don't feel quite comfortable in the role of mother either?

The first step toward understanding is an open dialogue. There is power in it. So let's look at some of the critical issues most applicable to adjusting from the full-time workforce to the part-time or stay-at-home world.

From Office to Home
Issue One: Am I Still an Equal Partner?

Although our spouses assure us that our job is the "hardest job in the world" and that they have "all the respect in the world for the job we do," let's face it: In the deepest recesses of our minds (and sometimes not so deep) we can sometimes feel that our role is not as important as that of being the breadwinner. (Not hard to imagine when it seems all we do all day is set the table, clear the table, feed the baby, change the baby, and so forth.) We start to question our worth in the relationship. We start questioning every purchase. We begin to ask for our spouse's input on decisions that we once made by ourselves. Our confidence begins to ebb.

Some of these questions come to us immediately after leaving a job. Some of them come after a few years. The questions develop into personal habits and before you know it, you can be strung out on anti-depressants and debating whether or not to go to Target lest you go over your purchasing limit!

This question of worth and value may be the number one issue you encounter as a housewife. Your importance as a stay-at-home mom or housewife is undeniable. Consider these thoughts if you're struggling with the idea that you may not be an equal partner.

* You both make the difference.
* Marriage is a partnership.
* Your role is *vital* to your family's success.
* You are a *partner* to your spouse.
* You are *both essential* to the success of your family.
* No one role is more important than the other.

The lawyers in the divorce case I mentioned and the members of Oprah's audience had it wrong. The fact is, you *are* vital to your husband's career success. He provides financial support, and your support enables him to stay late at work, leave home in the morning at the crack of dawn, and travel when necessary at will. Your support enables him to explore his career with complete freedom. You handle the household, meal preparation, nutrition, laundry, and childcare

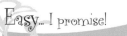

Easy... I promise!

Your time at home is not a day off from work. It took a long time before that concept sunk in for me.

for your family — and you do it all free of charge. Never downplay your role in your family. You are a critical element in its success.

Issue Two: Society's View of Stay-at-Home Moms

As the months of being an at-home mom progressed and I started to examine this new world of the at-home mom, I felt a little like one of those talk show hosts who would wear a fat suit to research how overweight people are treated in the world. I noticed people staring at me in the mall, wearing jeans in the middle of the day. Their stares seemed to say, "Why isn't she working? She's very spoiled. I would love to be able to lounge around in the middle of the day!"

Then every once in a while, a comment or two would creep into conversations with my working-mom counterparts about how "lucky" I was to stay at home. The adjective "easy" also started to enter the conversation when discussing life at home. I began to notice that women who are at-home feel the need to defend their role as stay-at-home mom.

How did we get to the point where we need to defend the decision to stay at home and care for our own children? Well, it wasn't overnight. Our generation is unique. We made money and had careers first, then we had children. Somehow society got the idea that women have a *choice* whether or not to go back to work. The reality of this choice is suspect. Many mothers have no choice, they must return to work. Other moms find that they must leave the workforce since the cost of daycare would outpace their paycheck. Regardless of the reality of the mom's situation, prevailing opinion is that if a woman stays home she has made a choice to bow out of the workforce for something easier. The realization that some people think this way can be difficult for the at-home mother to accept. It can make her resentful, confused, and wary of her choice. It can also make her just plain mad.

The irony is that none of the women of this generation remember signing on for this. The truth is that the evolution of the "role" of housewife has been a long time coming. For some perspective, let's look at the history of housewife through the most popular media of our generation's lives: the television.

Our generation had these women as TV role models of motherhood:

* Clair Huxtable from *The Cosby Show* — The successful lawyer working mother of six who seemed to be able to do it all, with ne'er a nanny around.

* Elise Keaton from *Family Ties* — The successful architect working mother of three who went "back" to work at a certain point but never had to hire a cleaning woman.

* Maggie Seaver from *Growing Pains* — A reporter working mother who managed family and career with

the help of her psychiatrist husband who worked from home.

If our mothers were watching TV for role models, which they probably were not, they would have found these women exemplifying the roles of the day:

* June Cleaver from *Leave It to Beaver* — A stay-at-home mom.

* Margaret Anderson from *Father Knows Best* — A stay-at home mom.

It's clear that society's views on what a mother should be able to do are exemplified in these TV moms. What a change. How did that happen? Let's look to the real people for guidance — our own mothers and the mothers of their generation.

Many of our mothers stayed home with us. If they worked, they worked part-time or after their youngest entered first grade. If they went to college, they did not have time to use their degree before starting a family. Many got pregnant early in their marriage. They stayed home with their children because it was expected. How did these women feel about the role of housewife? Betty Friedan in her 1963 book, *The Feminine Mystique*, describes the feeling this way:

> [It was] a strange stirring, a sense of dissatisfaction, a yearning that women suffered in the middle of the twentieth century in the United States. As she made the beds, shopped for groceries, matched slipcover material, ate peanut butter sandwiches with her children, chauffeured Cub Scouts and Brownies, and lay beside her husband at night she was afraid to ask even of herself the silent question — "Is this all?"[3]

That doesn't sound like our mothers were having a lot of fun, does it? Not that Friedan was speaking for every woman in America, but it struck a chord with enough women that it motivated them to unite and change things for themselves and for the daughters that would come after them.

And so, in my opinion, we have the previous generation of women to thank for ensuring that we would have "choices." The equal rights that women of our generation take for granted (so much so that we rarely even think about them) were hard fought. The ideals like entrance into college, the right to play women's sports in high school and college, the right to compete for jobs without discrimination based on gender, and equal pay for equal work were not widely held in our mother's generation. We should be grateful.

The women of this previous generation who bravely fought for these rights had one wish for the women who came after them, specifically that they would have choices for their future. To achieve this dream would mean their daughters would get to go to college if they so choose. Opportunities (whether we chose to accept them or not) are there for us. Entrance into the job market in any area that we wished to compete was also there for us. Truly amazing!

> Talk to your baby as you go about your day together. There's no reason to use baby talk. Of course, the drawback is you just might create a kid who never stops talking! But the impact on their speech development and vocabulary can only be positive.

The women who feel they need to justify their role as at-home parent or working parent need only to look at our history lesson for validation. More simply put, the women of this generation have been there, done that; we should answer to no one but ourselves. The women who have gone before us have provided us with the choices. We embraced the opportunities and have succeeded in the experiences that those choices provided for us. Again, the women of this generation answer to no one.

Keep a few things in mind when you feel like others are judging your decision.

* The only person's opinion that matters in this decision to stay home or to work is yours because you are the one who has to live it. If what you are doing makes you happy, that's all you need. No other barometer is necessary. This is an important life lesson on the parenting journey. Don't worry about what other people think.

* Most people in society who make comments about the stay-at-home mom are ignorant. I don't mean ignorant in the mean sense, I mean it in the literal sense. Anyone who hasn't stayed home with children doesn't know how difficult it is. You can't know anything until you actually do it, right? Try not to take the comments to heart. Someday, the women who make comments will be in your shoes and will be cursing themselves that they ever said anything so insensitive. So let it go in one ear and out the other and say to yourself, "Someday they will see."

* The decision to stay home or to work doesn't have to be an all-or-nothing decision. If you want to stop working for a while, work part-time, or stop working all together, remember that you are never locked into one deci-

sion. What is right for you at this point may not be right for you forever.

* When you hear someone say that the at-home mom/housewife has it easy, remember that the decision to leave a career is never an easy one. What many women feel when they leave a full-time job to care for their children is *relief*. Not relief because they have chosen the easy way out but because they have traded in two jobs for one.

> **As your baby grows, consider a simple bedtime routine. First a bath, then a bottle, and then reading a book is a common routine for settling down. Then put your baby down drowsy, but awake!**

* Most importantly, remember, if you choose to stay home for a while, you are not "wasting" an education or life experience but celebrating what the women who went before us wanted so desperately for us — a choice!

Issue Three: You're So Lucky!

I know you've heard this one. How could you not? It's everywhere. The sentiment that you're so lucky to be at home is more pervasive than a story on Britney Spears!

Don't believe me? Try an experiment. Ask any new mother who is staying home with her baby how she likes being home and the first thing out of her mouth will be, "I feel very lucky to be able to stay home with my child."

And a new mom does feel lucky. You have a healthy baby

and you are home taking care of him. The problem is that after months or years of hearing how lucky you are, resentment can start to grow. Or to put it more frankly, "If one more person tells me how lucky I am, I'm going to punch him out!"

Why might you feel resentment? It's simple. Motherhood is hard — really, really hard. To do the job 24/7 and constantly hear how lucky you are to do it takes something away from all the effort you put into being a mother. Moms are human, after all.

> Easy... I promise!
>
> **Make it a point to think the best of other mothers – especially those who have made different choices from you. Your choice is your choice. Hers is hers. Leave it that way.**

What human being wants to put so much effort into any endeavor without some feedback? No one. But as Ann Crittenden bemusedly points out in her book, *The Price of Motherhood*: "Your work on behalf of other family members is a labor of love, and we all know that love is its own reward."[4] So where does this leave a new mom who has decided or may decide to stay home with her new baby? Well, it often leaves her frustrated and alone.

I believe there are ways to change this "lucky" sentiment. Changing the "lucky" rhetoric might be a start. Words are powerful. If someone asks you how you like being home with your newborn, why not try the old Army slogan? Say, "It's the hardest job I'll ever love!" instead of "I'm so lucky."

Guilt – The Common Ground

I have been a working mom (working full-time outside the home) and a stay-at home mom.

My experience has been that the job of staying home is definitely harder than working full-time outside the house. To be completely responsible for another human being (or beings) while trying to get housework done is a never-ending, back-breaking, frustrating job. It simply cannot be compared to working in an office where you can actually concentrate on one thing at a time while sipping a cup of freshly brewed coffee (made by someone else).

On the other hand, the working mother has it hard because she automatically has *two* jobs. She has to get up and get the kids to daycare, get the kids home from daycare, make dinner, get the kids bathed, and do everything that the at-home mom may have a chance to do during the day. I kind of like to look at it like this: the at-home mom can spread out her energy throughout the entire day — if she is lucky. (Oops, I used my own bad word.) The working mom has to go full-force from the time she wakes up until the time she goes to bed. She has to be "on" all day.

While mentally the at-home mom is burnt out by being asked a million times a day the "mom" question or listening to "Mom, Mom, Mom, Mom, Mom" as she tries to get *one* thing done, the working mom is feeling pulled in a dozen directions. She probably has work from her job to finish at home, housework that needs to be done, and children to feed. She feels she is not doing any of it well. She has to juggle the babysitters, schoolwork, doctor's appointments, housework, and office work. The at-home mom does not have the outside work pressure, but she has the pressure of knowing that she has been home all day and has not been able to get a thing done in the house, and that her work experience is dwindling in value by the day, and her pension is growing at a rate of 0 percent.

What the two moms have in common is the guilt they both feel. The working mom feels guilt because she is not home with her child *and* because she can't stay late at work. The at-home mom feels guilt because she, too, feels she is not spending enough time with the kids because she is too busy preparing meals, cleaning up from meals, doing laundry, cleaning toilets,

> Easy... I promise!
>
> **When you and your husband resume sex after your baby's birth, don't forget to use birth control. Remember that it's possible to get pregnant before you have your first period!**

helping with homework, and grocery shopping — *and* she's not contributing to the family bank account. Isn't it ironic? The working mom feels the at-home mom has it made because she can spend time with the kids while the at-home mom feels guilt for exactly that reason — she doesn't feel she is spending enough time with the kids.

The working mom may feel the at-home mom is lucky because she can clean during the day. In truth, while working mom is sending her kids to daycare and leaving her house the way it is, the at-home mom is simply following her children around trying to clean up the messes that have been made while she has been home with them.

The at-home mom may think the working mom has it made because she has not had to pull her hair out all day dealing with children. In fact, the working mom has to run home after dealing with coworkers all day to deal with kids between the hours of 5:00

and 8:00 p.m., which each of us knows are the longest and most stressful hours of the day. Both moms have the "husband no-sex guilt" because both are too tired from working all day.

By now you may be noticing I haven't really answered the question, and you're right: The answer to the question is that there is no answer. Both are hard. One is not harder than the other. In fact, it is interesting to note how much the at-home mom and the working mom have in common, surely more than they differ.

I'd like to hold on to that concept for a while. The working mom and the at-home mom are more alike than they are different. They both have jobs, they are both exhausted, they both work hard, they both feel guilt that they are not doing a good enough job, they are both trying their best, and they are both trying to figure out an easier way. My sincere hope is that in the future both will start to focus on the concerns they have in common. I'm convinced with this focus, solutions will follow for all mothers.

Be Honest with Yourself

Changing the rhetoric about the topic of working moms and staying at home is crucial. The next step is to talk to other women. With talking comes understanding, empathy, and maybe even change.

It is so important to understand the reasons behind your choice to work outside the house or to stay at home and to be honest about them. It may be even more important to realize that you always have a choice. This is the true wish that our mothers had for us: to do what we truly believe is our mission in life without prejudice or regret!

Summary

Becoming a mother is one of those experiences that has been written about in sitcoms, movies, and books from generation to generation. Each generation of moms has a different "take" on the experience. For our generation of women, the overwhelming sentiment is that being a mom is an honor and supposed to make a woman feel complete. In addition, the opportunity for a woman to stay at home and raise her babies is to be particularly treasured. Be that as it may, for the moms who are home, in the trenches, doing the work, that sentiment can cause a great deal of frustration. This is because in other people's minds the hard work she does is eclipsed by what is seen as the ultimate gift of "being able to stay home." Fighting this sentiment seems so ungrateful, yet the lack of help, respect, or joy we feel in this role makes fighting an imperative. Using some of the tips in this chapter may help. Change your dialogue, ask for help when you need it, talk to your spouse or partner about the sacrifices you are making, and most important, be honest with yourself about your choices.

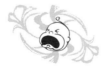

Chapter
Twelve

The Most Frustrating Job on the Planet

ell, we've looked a bit at the modern history of housewifery, but we haven't looked at the nuts and bolts of
the job. If this sounds a bit too dull for you or you think
it doesn't pertain to you because you work full-time, you might consider this fact: "The difference between the domestic workloads of
husbands with employed wives and husbands with unemployed
wives was found to be exactly ten minutes a day."[1] Either way,
you're doing housework or paying someone to do it. And if you're
doing any housework, then tips for streamlining the workload are
always welcome.

The Adjustment

Being at home, whether experienced earlier in your motherhood or
later in your motherhood, is an adjustment. This adjustment is not
yours alone; it is an adjustment for the whole family, particularly

for your husband. If you decide to stay at home with your baby, there will likely be a lengthy period of adjustment for you *and* for your husband. Some husbands seem to think that their at-home wife will magically take on the attributes of Cinderella, Mary Poppins, Julia Child, and Scarlett Johansson.

In the nutshell, his expectations may be that the house will be cleaner than ever; the kids will be freshly pressed, entertained, stimulated, and well-behaved; there will be freshly cooked gourmet meals every evening; and you will serve them in your red teddy. (Okay, maybe not serve them in your red teddy but have the red teddy at the ready to pull out at the appropriate time.)

Ask any husband whether he feels this way and he may fib. Many will not own up to it. They know the politically correct response, but in the quiet recesses of their minds they have a certain expectation of how wonderful it will be to have a stay-at-home wife. This expectation is in itself a puzzle. This is the same guy who shared in all of the chores when you were first married and did so with no problem when you were holding down a full-time job. What's changed? Expectations.

You are no longer working, you see, so in his mind you now have time to handle all these other jobs in addition to caring for your new baby. Even if he knows how tough things are with an infant because he's been home with you, he may still expect

> *Easy... I promise!*
>
> **It's never too early to start reading books to your baby. Board books are sturdy and their text is short. Choose rhyming and sing-song type books for your infant or ones that focus on one vivid picture per page.**

some of these other perks. When you ask him why he suddenly expects all these other things to be done, he may say — now brace yourself — "Because it's your job." Ah, the dreaded "because it's your job" comment. What is horrible about this revelation is that you may be thinking the same thing yourself. Although you'd never admit it out loud, you may be thinking, *Isn't this my job now? Why can't I get it all done?*

After a few weeks, you'll try to explain that taking care of the baby takes all your time and that you don't have time for much else. It will do no good. He's been swept up in a tidal wave of societal sentiment that has carried him far away from the domestic shore. Keep in mind that his coworkers are patting his back, congratulating him on enabling his wife to stay home with his child. He hears this everyday. He's brainwashed and he's confused.

Let's look at the facts. You are no longer bringing in any money. You are at home all day. This is what you wanted to do, to stay at home to raise your child. From his standpoint, there's got to be something in it for him. But the reality is that instead of life getting easier for him, it's actually going to get harder. He's still going to have to pitch in with the housework. There's less money coming in. He's now *the* financial provider for the household. And he has to come home to a postpartum wife who is going to hand him a screaming infant the second he walks in the door after working a full day. Add to this all the societal pressure he is feeling to connect with his child, be empathetic to his wife — and don't even think about mentioning sex, you insensitive clod. What exactly is he supposed to get out of this deal?

New fathers need to be eased into the realty of the new situation. This is a tough one. The women who have the most success are the ones who involve their husbands in the process every step of the way. Help him understand by sharing the following affirmations with him:

* Having one of us stay home to raise the children is a conscious decision that we are making because we think it has value for the future of our children and our marriage.

* We are ready to make some sacrifices in order to achieve these goals.

* The sacrifices will include not having a perfectly clean house all the time and not having gourmet dinners every night. (This goes for women as well as men. I've known many a woman who would shift that "perfectly clean" house expectation to her husband because she would be too tired to do it and guilt him into doing it. He's tired too, remember!)

* When we see our baby fed and safe in bed each night we will consider our job to be done for the day.

* We will try to be considerate of each other's needs during this time and try not to put added pressure on each other. This includes resuming a protected sex life when appropriate.

Educating your spouse on the realities of the "at-home" world is your first mission and the mission that you must continue to work toward each day.

The Nuts and Bolts of the Job

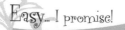

Once you are a little more comfortable with the role of new mommy you will have to face the reality of housework. I hesitate to even write this. How do I get around sounding like some present-day Miss Manners? Do I denigrate the successful women

> **As a mom, you are only as happy as your saddest child.**

of today by suggesting that they need to learn something as simple as housework? No way! Am I suggesting that there is a need for the return of the home economic classes that we spurned for advanced physics and tech school back in high school? Absolutely not!

However, I realize that it doesn't do anybody any good to pretend that housework and cleaning is not an issue for women. The fact is that cleaning, laundry, and grocery shopping have to get done. Some fortunate souls pay someone to attend to some of these tasks, but the majority of families in this country do their own cleaning and cooking. It's a fact of life and after you have kids the task becomes even more challenging. My best advice is to come up with a plan that enables you to spend as little time as possible doing it.

Let's face it. Our mothers raised us to be independent, to go to school, to get an education, to have a career. We were too busy being involved in activities, sports, and college to watch and learn from our mothers how to be a housewife. Yet that's just what we need to know about as we raise our families. How do we do it if we never learned it? Why do you think there are such successful shows as *Mission Organization*? Because we never learned how to handle housework and raising children!

The first rule of housekeeping and the most helpful one is the art of the pick-up. Through the years I've actually encountered women who appear to have a perpetually clean house. Eventually I had to ask them how they do it, and they revealed the secret. The secret is that their houses are not always truly clean. The fact that the house looks clean is just an illusion. I knew it. It's impossible to do this job without the use of magic. This magic comes in the form of the pick-up.

Quite simply, if you keep your house picked up at all times, it looks clean, even if it

Easy... I promise!

In my area, it costs about $80 to pay someone to clean your house. If you have it done every other week (okay, that's what I do), that's $40 a week. That's equivalent to one take-out dinner for the two of you. It's worth it, don't you think?

isn't. The added bonus of the picked-up house is that when you finally have time to clean something, you can get right down to the cleaning without having to do the hour long pick-up first! Picking up is always the best place to start, too. Just start putting things away. The more organized an area is, the clearer your head becomes and the more ready you will be to deal with the tasks at hand.

The Circus Act

They say everything changes after a baby. "They" are right. Even doing the simplest chores can seem like a humongous feat — a juggling act, in fact. The trick to getting things done with a new baby is to start to look at the process differently. Instead of having blocks of time to get tasks done, you now have slivers of time. You have to learn to take tasks apart.

> **Easy... I promise!**
>
> **Lower your expectations of yourself if you need to. No mom can do things perfectly. No house can always be clean.**

Instead of cleaning the whole kitchen, for example, you now may get five minutes to empty the dishwasher. Instead of cleaning the whole bathroom, you may get a chance to scrub the toilet. This can be a tough adjustment to make, especially if you are used to getting all your cleaning done in one shot. I remember one couple in our first neighborhood. They loved their house to be spotless and Friday was their cleaning night. They would get a six-pack of beer (pre-children, of course) and clean the house from top to bottom every Friday night. After a newborn, those days were gone.

It is helpful to separate any job into smaller tasks that you can return to throughout the day. For example, if you always have your laundry separated à la the compartment hamper, you've eliminated the separating step when you have a minute to do a load of laundry. Being able to do a little bit of work at a time is a valuable skill. When my first was born, I can remember asking my neighbor, a veteran mother of four, "How will I get anything done with this baby needing me all the time?" She noticed that the baby was lying happily on the floor looking at his toys. She said, "There you go. You've got five minutes before he starts crying to empty the dishwasher." I thought, "Woohoo, five whole minutes!" Get used to it. I did. Now I multitask to the point where I always have at least four or five things going at a time, as do most mothers I know. Multitasking is real!

Even with multitasking you may find that you are still having trouble getting things done. Some have found that getting a house cleaner once every two weeks is an enormous help. It can be a great relief to know that at least two times a month the toilets and bathrooms will be really clean. Of course, it's not easy to afford that on one income. Furthermore, a house cleaner may not be the answer to your prayers that you think it is. All the daily stuff and maintenance will still need to be done. So, beware! If you hire one you might think that your house will be spotless all the time. Remember, the house cleaner is not going to put all your stuff away, do your laundry, put the clothes away, go grocery shopping, cook, or pay the bills. (If only we all had an "Alice" like the *Brady Bunch* had!) If it is understood that the house cleaner is there to make sure at least twice a month the bathrooms get a thorough cleaning, things get dusted, and the floors get done, great! Go for it! Most families find this expense prohibitive, however, or they prefer to spend their disposable income on other things. One idea to consider is hiring one for a period of time, like the first few months after the baby's birth.

Random Cleaning Tips

In addition to the pick-up, I have some hard and fast tips that I have come across over the years. Take this as a little friendly advice from someone who's been in the trenches for a while.

* If you have the time, do it. You may not have the time later. Doing the pots and dishes is a great example. How often do you tell yourself you'll do it tomorrow and when tomorrow comes you end up with something more important to do?

* Get as much done the night before as you can — dish-

es, bottles prepared, diapers stocked, and so forth. Never put off until tomorrow what you can do today! Now I know I have heard that one before. Oh yes, good ol' Ben Franklin!

> Easy... I promise!
>
> **If you're exhausted, don't forget to nap when you can. Cleaning and laundry can wait. Groceries usually can too.**

* When making a decision regarding what to keep and what to throw away consider whether the item is for your life as you live it today. If you don't use it or look at it at this time in your life, throw it away. Do not keep things because you think you may need them some day. If you actually do need it, buy it again. The money you might save is not worth the aggravation of the clutter — and that's assuming you'd actually be able to find the item when you need it.

* They say that the tools make the man — or the woman as the case may be. Invest in a good bucket, good paper towels (not the kind that come apart when they get wet), a good-sized duster, and a decent broom.

* Always start a bedroom with making the bed. Once the bed is made, progress seems to have already begun!

* *Always* clean your kitchen before you go to bed. It's a lot less stressful to come down in the morning to a clean kitchen. Starting the day with yesterday's dirty dishes is so depressing.

Bathrooms

Try to clean the bathrooms once a week. If you stay on top of it, it will be a fifteen-minute job instead of an hour job. Here's how to do it quickly:

* Sweep.
* Use a paper towel to clean the mirror.
* Squirt the toilet and the sink and the counter top with "scrubbing bubbles," and sprinkle cleaner into the toilet.
* Wipe down the toilet with a paper towel and scrub the inside of the toilet bowl with a brush.
* Wipe down the counter top and the sink. Rinse the paper towel, wipe it down again, and you are done.
* Use the paper towel that you cleaned the sink with to wipe the floor around the toilet.
* To clean the floor every other week get an old towel, immerse in soapy water in the bathtub, and rinse out.
* Wrap the towel around a sponge mop and mop the floor.
* Wipe around the sides of the floor with another old towel.
* When you're finished, throw the towels in the laundry and wash them.

Odd Jobs

Motherhood and housekeeping are all about odd jobs! Here are some tips for some of those.

* *Keep a standard grocery list of items you purchase each week.* My mother used to keep a grocery list in her computer with the basics — bread, milk, butter, eggs, and so forth. She would print off a new list every week and add to it for the week, which saved her a lot of tedious writing of the same items every week.

* *Write your grocery list in the order of the grocery store aisles.* This really does take time off your trip. Also, try to place the items on the conveyor belt in the order they will be put away at home (frozen foods together, lunchmeats and refrigerated items together, canned goods together, and so forth). The key here is to save as much time as you can.

* *As for dinner, the trick is to cook the kind of dinners that will last you at least two nights.* Then sprinkle in some sandwiches and a take-out pizza and you are done for the week.

Here are some ideas for things that will last you two nights:

* *Bake a turkey breast or roast beef with some vegetables.* Both are great for leftovers; add biscuits to the second night's dinner or simply make turkey or roast beef sandwiches.

* *Cook lots of ground meat.* Use half one night for spaghetti and meat sauce and the other half for taco meat the next night. Remember cooked ground meat can be frozen and used later.

* *Cook a whole pack of chicken breasts.* Use half with vegetables and salad one night, and use the other half with salsa and cheese for a chicken salsa pizza (in a prepared pizza shell, of course).

* *Most experienced mothers swear the best way to handle laundry is to do a little bit each day.* I have *one* laundry hamper in my bedroom closet with three compartments.

* *Use baskets — and lots of them*. Organization — or the lack thereof — is a common problem for families. I have baskets everywhere. Buy some big ones to put under the sinks to keep your stuff from falling over.

Easy... I promise!

Remember that everything is a phase. It makes life with a baby so much more enjoyable. Savor the good times and remind yourself that the bad times will pass.

A Schedule for Mom?

You may know some women who like to use a daily schedule. I loved using a schedule for my babies, but for me? Not so much. I could never seem to get the hang of it. You know what I'm talking about. Laundry on Monday, groceries on Tuesdays, vacuuming on Wednesdays, and so forth. Many women find a schedule to be a useful tool though. Let's take a look at a schedule that my girlfriend's mom followed in the 60s.

6:00 – 6:30	Wake up and wash up
6:30 – 7:00	Wake up kids, make breakfast
7:00 – 7:15	Eat breakfast
7:15 – 7:30	Get dressed
7:30 – 8:30	Drive Dad to train station
8:30 – 12:30	Drive home, do errands on the way (if necessary), clean up kitchen, make beds, do laundry and clean bathrooms (each day), make dinner (to be heated up later)
12:30 – 1:00	Lunch
1:00 – 3:00	Sew (clothes/curtains/tablecloths/etc.), iron, or volunteer at school

3:00 – 3:30	Exercise
3:30 – 4:00	Nap
4:00 – 4:30	Shower and dress
4:30 – 5:00	Serve dinner
5:30 – 6:30	Pick up Dad from train station
6:30 – 10:00	Serve Dad dinner, entertain Dad, read newspaper or books, pray Rosary

Obviously, this mother's children were in school at this point, but it is still very interesting. A schedule for today's mother might look something like this:

7:00 – 7:15	Wake up, brush teeth
7:15 – 8:30	Get kids ready for school, encourage kids to get their own breakfast and make their lunches for school, take kids to school
9:00 – 10:30	Exercise at the YMCA
10:30 – 11:00	Shower
11:00 – 12:00	Start some laundry, make phone calls, grocery shop
12:00 – 12:30	Eat lunch
12:30 – 2:30	Pay bills; catch up on e-mail; Internet shop; keep laundry going; add all new play dates, parties, school functions to Palm Pilot.
2:30 – 5:00	Pick up kids, help kids with homework, drive kids to activities, and pick up kids from activities
5:00 – 7:00	Decide what to do for dinner (make it or order it), eat
7:00 – 8:00	Kids' baths and bed
8:00 – 10:00	Watch sitcoms, news with husband until bedtime

The glaring difference between the schedule from the 60s and one from today is the kids' "schedule." The 60s mom is not running around, carting her children everywhere. She also wasn't involved with the kids' homework. And this is a schedule for the "at-home" mom. Essentially, today's "at-home" mom has about 2.5 hours per day — unless she has volunteered for school or one of her kids is sick or someone has to get to a doctor's appointment — to do all of the

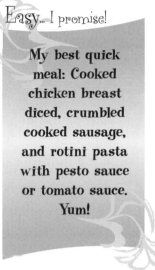

Easy... I promise!

My best quick meal: Cooked chicken breast diced, crumbled cooked sausage, and rotini pasta with pesto sauce or tomato sauce. Yum!

things to keep a household running. What about the working mom? How does she do it? Housework is a tough issue for all women. A "schedule" for mom may or may not be the answer.

Mom Always Said

When it comes to the housework, an important part of the new mother equation, just remember what my mother always told me. Your job first and foremost is the safety and well-being of your children. Housework is secondary and there will be days you just will not get to it. If you concentrate on keeping the bathrooms and the kitchen clean, you will be okay. Finding time to clean up the bathrooms and kitchen is just a part of providing a safe environment for your children to be in. The rest can wait. And wait and wait.

Summary

"Housewife" is something of a negative term, isn't it? No matter what you call it — domestic engineer, head of household, homemaker — the job is still the same. Essentially, we are the chief cook and bottle washers. I hope that this chapter has given you some ideas to make the job a bit easier, or better put, to reduce the amount of time you have to spend actually doing the job. Most importantly, I hope reading the chapter put a smile on your face, and gives you the strength to attack another day.

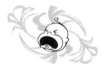

Chapter Thirteen

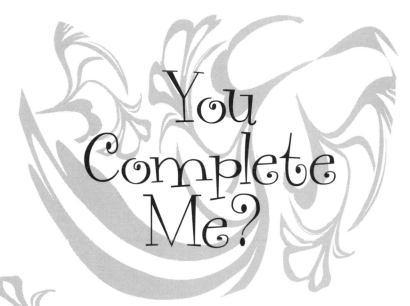

You Complete Me?

Have you ever wondered why you sometimes feel like your life isn't as complete as you thought it would be after becoming a mother? Well, Abraham Maslow would have something to say about that. Maslow, a twentieth century champion of humanistic psychology, developed the idea that each person is on a journey to self-actualization (or fulfillment). In turn there was, he believed, a hierarchy of needs that had to be met in order to achieve this self-actualization. Maslow said that those who have not achieved this self-actualization feel there is something missing, a feeling of not being complete. The hierarchy of needs is now not only used in psychology but also in management principles and techniques.

I believe Maslow's theory of self-actualization goes a long way to explaining why the at-home mother may feel depressed or that her life is somehow incomplete. This feeling is exacerbated by society's view of how "lucky" she should feel because she is at home with her children. Examining Maslow's theory and applying its findings to your own life can help you to understand your feelings and find your own path to self-actualization and happiness.[1]

According to Maslow, whether your needs are being fulfilled (and how they're being fulfilled) can go a long way toward explaining your behavior and ultimately your happiness. Maslow's hierarchy of needs looks like a pyramid. The lowest needs are basic needs — oxygen, food, and water. The next level of needs are security and safety needs; the third level of needs are social, including love, affection, and a sense of belonging; the fourth level of needs are esteem needs; and the fifth level of needs are for self-actualization and fulfillment.[2]

> **Easy... I promise!**
>
> **If you're feeling dissatisfied at home but you have no plans to go back to work anytime soon, consider a continuing education class. It's a great opportunity to meet new people, get out of the house, and learn something new. Your local community college probably offers loads of interesting courses.**

Once the lower (or basic) needs are all met (imagine a pyramid), then the "higher" needs need to be fulfilled for the person to be happy. In other words, once our bellies are full we crave comfort, once we have comfort we crave acceptance, once we have acceptance we crave self-actualization or "meaning in our lives." How are we contributing to the world? Are we reaching our full potential? If we are not, we are not happy. It stands to reason that if we are starving, we have little need to think beyond the basic need of food. We would spend little time pondering whether we have had an impact on another person or on the world for that matter. Some people never yearn beyond the first level of the pyramid.

What does this have to do with motherhood? Everything. When your baby is a newborn, your instinct is survival. The need for survival for you and for your baby is all you can think about on a day-to-day basis. Am I going to meet the needs of my baby today? When am I going to sleep again? Am I going to be able to do this tomorrow? Adjusting to having another human being completely dependent on you is overwhelming. The days and nights squish together. All the issues that you had before, like decorating your house, vacation planning, work issues, or other people's problems (issues that maybe your friends and family members now have), seem trivial.

The comedian Dana Carvey used to joke in his routine that shortly after he and his wife had a baby, his friends would call him and say things like, "I slept 'til noon and I'm still tired." Meanwhile Carvey and his wife "hadn't slept in weeks." That's survival mode.

And when you're in it, all the other needs you have for success in your job, fulfillment in your relationships, and so forth fly out the window as you struggle to catch up on sleep and keep this little person alive. This may last for months or even years at some level depending on how many children you have or whether you decide to stay home with your children.

I had my own experience with Maslow's hierarchy. When my son turned two and I had just quit my full-time job, it didn't take long for me to get frustrated being home. Caring for my son was never the problem. It was everything that went along with that. In a journal entry from April 1994 I wrote, "I do know that I want to be close to (my son) and that I do enjoy taking care of him. What I don't like is the housekeeping side of the issue." Of course I also hated giving up the money, security, pension, work experience, and freedom. I didn't like the reality that my "job" was to care for a home — a job that came with no money, no pension, and no evaluation. Cooking, cleaning, and caring for the house — yuck! I remember thinking, *Is this what I've become? Am I now to be measured by how clean my house is? Is getting three loads of laundry done in one day the measurement of my success?* I frequently had to remind myself that this is what I wanted, to raise children. Why wasn't I happy?

Easy... I promise!

Set aside some time to pursue your interests. Consider hiring a babysitter for even just a few hours a week so you can garden, read, paint, or shop!

These thoughts would plague me for a while and then another child would come along and I would not have time to think of such frivolous ideas. I was concerned about another life, when I would get some sleep — the basic needs on my pyramid. Then the baby would get a little older and the thoughts would come creeping back. The more I thought about it, the more I realized the truth: I *am* doing what I want to be doing, but I wanted to be doing other things, too. I remembered being at work and thinking of all the things I could be doing if I were home. Being with my son, yes, but also writing, exercising, reading, decorating — all things I had no energy to do by the time I got home from work.

I remembered all the guilt I felt at not being there to see and encourage my son's first steps, his first words, his first puzzle. I finally realized that I did have the control. If I wanted to do something I had to make it happen.

I realized that all my lower pyramid needs were met. I wasn't hungry. My relationship with my husband satisfied my need for love. I felt security thanks to the upbringing my parents gave me. But something was missing. For me it was the need to create, to express my views, to contribute to the outside world, to feel important. These are my self-actualization needs.

I started writing when I was a kid. I have notebooks going back to when I was nine. I also love to read. Doing these things makes me feel whole. The point is you must take that first step to find out what is going to help you achieve your self-actualization. Sometimes you won't even feel the need for it. That's okay. But at times you may not feel complete. At those times, you need to explore what will help you to feel fulfilled. It may be working outside the home, or exercising, or volunteering at the school or a local food bank.

If you need something more than motherhood to feel fulfilled, it's okay. Why shouldn't you be multifaceted? Your husband can be father, husband, friend, executive, handyman, and more. Why can't mothers wear many hats as well?

Just because you are immersed in the important task of raising human beings does not mean that you should lose sight of your individual needs. I was inspired by this quote from Martha Graham the first time I read it:

There is a vitality, a life force, an energy, a quickening that is translated through you into action: and because there is only one of you in all time, this expression is unique. If you block it, it will never exist through any other medium and it will be lost. The world will not have it. You must keep that channel open. It is not for you to determine how good it is nor how valuable, nor how it compares with other expressions. It is for you to keep it yours, clearly and directly.[3]

I recently met a forty-something woman at a mom's group. She had worked as an international marketing executive at a large corporation, but once she had a child, she decided that it was her job to stay home and take care of him. She quit her job and now was trying to keep up with her very active 18 month old. At the mom's group, I noticed her trying desperately to persuade the child to come in the house so she could enjoy a cup of coffee. She looked at me wearily and exclaimed, "Does anyone really *like* this?" "No!" I said, "no one really likes this."

> Easy... I promise!
>
> **Finding a babysitter is like finding a new job. It's all about the power of networking. Ask friends, family members, neighbors, coworkers, and message board friends for references. You'll be amazed the great leads that come back to you.**

Who enjoys chasing after a one-year-old who could hurt himself at any second, when all you want is a simple cup of coffee? We keep the secret, I told her, because we want to maintain membership in the club. What we do as mothers is important. We hope the sacrifices will have a positive impact on our children's present and future. *How* we do it is what is open for debate. I told her that if she was miserable staying home she should go back to work. If she is miserable, her son will sense that and be miserable. Why should she stay home and give up *her* career? Her husband didn't give up his.

Summary

The point is, having a child doesn't suddenly transform you. If you have always loved dancing, working, traveling, you always will. All those desires to succeed and compete and create do not fall out with the placenta! Continue doing what makes you feel whole, find a balance, and your child will respond. You can't change who you are in the hopes of being the kind of mother you think your child should have. This particular woman decided to go back to work with a limited scope to her position. Last I heard she was doing well and working hard to achieve balance in her life. Maslow would be proud!

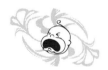

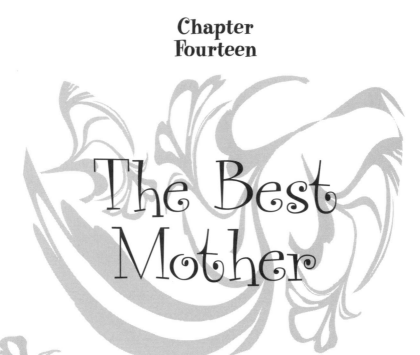

Chapter Fourteen

The Best Mother

When women are pregnant for the first time, they often wonder whether they'll possess the proper parenting instincts the moment the baby is born. The answer is yes *and* no. If only babies were born with instructions, then our parenting abilities might be flawless. I remember being in the hospital and thinking, *These people are crazy for letting me take this kid home.* I barely knew how to change a diaper.

My husband and I attended the "infant care" classes provided by the hospital after our first baby was born. It included instruction on bathing, changing, and feeding. (Note that we took the classes *after* the baby was born. This procrastination is a common phenomenon among first-time parents; the clinical term is *denial*.) One of the first things we learned in class was that if the baby had not finished his bottle within an hour, the formula must be thrown away. We had been desperately trying to feed our infant son the same bottle for about three hours. Oopsie! I couldn't believe we'd made a major mistake so quickly.

Mistakes aside, the question of how to be the best mother to our children is a question that seems to plague our generation the most. While the mothers of the past may have considered that question, the mothers of the Information Age seem to obsess about it. We are surrounded by books, TV shows, the Internet, professionals, and other mothers who criticize and question our every "mother move." The suggestions for good mothering in the twenty-first century run from homeschooling, to participating in a Mommy and Me class, to bonding with our children in utero. Where does the quest to be the perfect mother end? If I had the definitive answer to the conundrum I would be on a speaking tour for $100,000 a day plus expenses!

> Easy... I promise!
>
> **Treat finding a qualified babysitter outside your family as a number one priority. Family is always great in the case of an emergency, but a great babysitter will free you to take some time for yourself.**

Rather than looking to today's trends, I have learned to listen to the many words of wisdom passed down from my parents, grandparents, and great-grandparents. After all, they provided the schedule! Their insights have proven invaluable.

Their collective insight says to always remember that your children are lent to you for a time. You do not own them. They are individuals with their own hopes, dreams, personalities, and temperaments. As a parent, your job is first and foremost to raise them to set them free. You must raise them to deal with the unfairness in life as well as its rewards. All the rest of your parenting strategy should stem from the understanding that you are raising them to set them free. Consider this quote from Khalil Gibran's *The Prophet*. On the subject of children he writes:

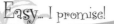

Easy... I promise!

Does your husband like to cook? Let him! Even if he doesn't, try to agree on splitting the cooking duties – unless you love to cook, of course.

> Your children are not your children. They are the sons and daughters of Life's longing for itself. They come through you but not from you, and though they are with you yet they belong not to you. You are the bows from which your children as living arrows are sent forth.[1]

Simply put, this says that you raise your children in such a way that they can leave you and function in the world without you. Your one and only job is to supply your children with the knowledge, experience, and wherewithal to be able to live without you *and* to be independent, useful members of society. What a task. Not only is it *not* easy, but it is fraught with perils and requires sacrifice and courage.

In an attempt to set your children free, there are three basic guidelines that I believe will keep you on the straight and narrow. Ironically, only *one* of them is directly related to your children.

1. Take care of yourself.
2. Take care of your spouse.
3. Learn how to say no to your children.

Take Care of Yourself

The first and most important step to setting your children free is to take care of yourself. When you are the primary caregiver, it is easy to forget that you even have needs. Motherhood is a 24 hour a day proposition. Children's needs are overwhelming, so why are *your* needs so important as you raise them? Your needs are important for the same reason that a flight attendant tells you to put your oxygen mask on first and then to see to your child in the case of an emergency. You need to be cared for in order to be able to care for your child.

When your needs always take the backburner, your mood and state of mind will be affected. Namely, resentment may trickle down to each member of your family. This affects not only how they interact with you, but also how they interact with each other. Over the years, this can have some serious consequences to your relationship with your husband and your family overall. It does not pay to sacrifice your happiness for the happiness of the family because they will sense you are unhappy and they will be unhappy as well. Conversely, when you make time for yourself, it pays off in the increased stability of your family. In addition, addressing your own needs forces you to let your family fend for themselves a bit. Over time, this forced independence helps your children to become more self-sufficient. You will have succeeded in enabling your children to take care of themselves.

> Easy... I promise!
>
> **If you have time for nothing else, at least make time to take a shower. Put the baby in a bouncy seat on the bathroom floor, play peek-a-boo with the shower curtain if you have to, but take the few minutes to make yourself feel refreshed.**

If you're a mother for the first time with a newborn baby, this may sound crazy. How could you possibly think of anything but your baby's needs at this time? This thought process is understandable. You are focused on the baby and the baby's needs and rightly so. At this point you probably can't imagine a time when you can think about yourself again. But I promise you, the baby will grow!

As she starts to grow and you start to feel more comfortable with motherhood, try to think of yourself in little ways. Before you know it, your baby will be able to pull herself up, fall asleep on her own, and roll over. As you see these changes taking place, remind yourself that as your child gets older she can be more independent and that it is okay to start to remember your own needs. What needs should a new mother begin to think about? Let's start with the personal needs that go by the wayside after a baby is born.

I bet I can name the first personal errand that goes out the window once a woman has a baby. It's like an episode of *Family Feud*. "We asked 100 women, what is the first errand to go out the window when you have a baby?" Survey says: "Going to the hair salon." Ding, ding, ding! Why do so many give up on the hair after the birth of a baby? The answer is because a hair appointment is the one personal errand that takes the longest, takes you out of the house, and seems frivolous. It's not like grocery shopping after all. I know women who have gone months after having a baby without getting their hair done.

Strange, isn't it? Your hair is the one personal feature that is most obvious to you. You look in the mirror every day and you can't avoid seeing it. Ironically, just when you start to feel like yourself again after the birth, you begin to not look like yourself! Perhaps you feel guilty for leaving the baby so early in life for a two-hour hair appointment. I implore you, don't put it off. After the two-week post-partum time is up and you can drive, schedule an appointment. As silly as this might sound, one of the first steps in being a good mom may be to make a hair appointment.

Likewise, when you wake up in the morning, don't put off taking a shower. If the baby is screaming, let him scream. Keep him in the safety of his crib or put him in a bouncy seat on the floor while you shower. He'll be just fine. Everything starts to look better after you have that shower. Also, if you are in the habit of putting make-up on, take the five minutes to continue to do it.

> Easy... I promise!
>
> **If someone offers help (doing your laundry or dishes, cleaning your bathroom, making a dinner), say, "Yes, thank you," and let them do it! You can do the same for someone else someday, and your reward will be how much they appreciate it, because you have been there!**

These are just a few examples of how you can continue to think about your personal needs once the baby is born. Later, as the baby grows you can start to think about some of the other areas of your life that you may want to explore. For example, you may have been considering going back to school or taking a night course or learning a new skill. The point is, do not put off your dreams because you have a child. It's important, even if you focus on just one new thing.

Remember, if you have interests outside the needs of your family, pursuing them helps your family be more self-sufficient. Having other interests that make you happy gives your life balance and will give your family members a sense of responsibility and pride in their accomplishments due to their new-found independence. It's important to realize that you are not only teaching your children how to behave, but you are also teaching them how to be a parent. As hard as it is, someday you will have to set them free to make their own choices out in the world. Do *not* put your life on hold until they reach 18. A girlfriend once told me that when you have children, they should learn to adjust to *your* schedule, not the other way around. Furthermore, consider that your children are an addition to your family and not the center of it, which brings us to our next rule.

Take Care of Your Spouse

In addition to putting yourself last, you may also be tempted to put your spouse last (okay, maybe second to last). But remember, your spouse is your family, too — the first member of your family as a matter of fact. He, too, is going through a change. He now has to share you. Many men worry about the change in relationship with their spouse after the birth of a baby.

Aside from the immediate worries of a new mouth to feed, they probably have a heightened sense of the change in relationship with their spouse, both sexually and otherwise. Talk to him about these issues. Be forthcoming about the information that is going to be important to him — namely, when you feel you might be able to resume sex. As cliché as it may seem, sex is going to be foremost in his mind. Getting some alone time with him may help to get sex foremost in your mind as well. Plan some alone time with him to get you in the mood. Don't put off dating until the baby turns one. Let your husband know you are willing to spend a few hours away from the baby to spend time with him.

Your relationship with your husband is exceedingly important because a healthy marriage is the best gift you can give your children. Being around two people who love and respect each other provides genuine security for children. Furthermore, remember that you are teaching your child how to be a good spouse. He will learn from watching you and your husband how to treat his future spouse and how a spouse should be treated — so put your spouse first.

Now this doesn't mean that you ignore your baby to meet your husband's needs. It *does* mean if the man wants to sit with you that maybe you sit with him instead of cleaning the bathroom. The bathroom will wait, your relationship with your husband won't. It *does* mean that you try *not* to bring your infant into bed with you. Commandment Number Six as described in Chapter Seven clearly states, "thou shalt not bring the baby into bed with you." The bed is what you share with your husband. It is your private space to do the things that husbands and wives do. Bringing your baby into this dominion tells your husband that he is *not* number one anymore. It *does* mean that you let the baby cry for a bit in the middle of the night (after approximately three months) to help get him back to sleep. Try to remember that you are married to your husband, not the baby. The baby is going to grow and leave you, but your husband is going to be around for the rest of your life.

Now, in order to ensure your children actually *do* leave, you must follow the third guideline and learn to say no to your children.

Learn to Say No

In the movie *A Bronx Tale*, the mob boss is speaking with a teenager who idolizes him. The teenager asks, "Is it better for a person to be feared or loved?" The mob boss replies, "It's nice to be both, but I would rather be feared." Substitute "feared" for "respected" and you have the game-winning answer to how to be the best parent. Insist on respect from your children and the good behavior will follow. Without the respect, you might as well pack it in. With this in mind, there are many situations that will test your resolve in the quest for respect. The first and most important test will be in your ability to say no to your children.

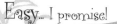

Easy... I promise!

Trust your instincts. Always. When it comes to your kids, listen to that little voice inside yourself.

Saying no is one of the hardest things for parents to do. It's really very unfair. Children come into your life completely dependent on you. They are helpless little creatures who need you for everything, and in the beginning you have to do everything for them. Soon you get used to doing everything for them and calming them as they scream and cry. Your goal is to make them happy and content. Then, before your know it, you have to require them to do things by themselves and make them unhappy by saying no. It seems the ultimate contradiction. But "no" could be the most important word in your parenting vocabulary.

It is my theory that saying no when appropriate is *the* way to command respect from your children. With respect comes functioning, happy, productive individuals. In order to prove my thesis, I invite you to join me for a trip through the future. We'll begin about the time your child starts to walk.

You and your toddler are on a play date. All the toddlers are clinging to their mothers for the first five minutes, but then they start to get adventurous. They start to explore. Suddenly, your child has reached the television set. Now, he is in no immediate danger (I think we can all agree that saying no when a child in danger is easy) because the TV is on a TV stand with no chance of toppling over. However, you notice the owner of the house getting antsy. In response to this situation you:

A. Do nothing. The owner of the house must realize that these are children and children will be children — they are made to explore.

B. Immediately get up and physically move your toddler away from the TV, saying, "No" while you do it.

C. From your position on the floor say, "Don't touch that."

I think you can probably guess that my answer to this question would be B. In fact, for as many times as your toddler would go to the TV to touch it, I would have you get up each and every time to tell the toddler, "No." This might mark the end to your foray into the play date world (you can bet I didn't go out too much), but it is important to show your child that you are in charge and that respecting other things and more importantly, you, is lesson number one. This lesson can't start soon enough. In addition, your "respect bucket "will begin to fill up. A respect bucket is the imaginary container of the amount of respect your children have for you.

Let's take a look at the other answers and the effects they might have. Answer A would be the easiest answer. After all, you are tired, the baby is not in any danger, and the play date is supposed to be a break for you, right? But how's that respect bucket looking? Empty. Answer C seems like a good answer but this solution can be confusing to the toddler. "What exactly is Mommy saying not to touch?" Also, "Mommy's not getting up to tell me not to touch it like she did when I went to touch the oven, so it must not be that big a deal." How's your respect bucket looking now? Could be about half full.

You may think that touching a TV is not such a big deal, so

why all the fuss? Your handling of the touching of the TV is a test. It is important to address this behavior early and whenever you see it. Respecting other people's things and calling your child on it is an important step and one that you will be tested on again and again and again. When you see a behavior that you do not like, you need to address it the moment it happens and every time after that in order for the right behavior to become hard-coded. It's no easy task. Why do you think there are so many messed up kids running around? All you have to do is to watch *Supernanny* to see that the kids are running the homes. The reason it happens is because it's much harder to address bad behavior at the time it happens. It is much easier to put up with it, pretend we don't see, or just hope it will go away, in the short-term at least.

My parents once told me that children are essentially formed by the time they are seven. I don't know who said it originally, but I believe it. With that in mind, you must keep close track of the important behaviors that children exhibit early in their life and address them. There is no *later*. If you address what you see now, it may not be an issue later.

But let's continue on our trip into the future. Your child is now a little older. You're in the grocery store and your child is in the cart. She's old enough to recognize candy in the check-out line. She's pointing and indicating that she wants some candy. It's an hour before dinner. There's a long line of restless people behind you. How do you handle the situation?

    A. You give the toddler the candy. It's just some candy after all.

    B. You say, "No, we are having dinner soon."

    C. You give the child something else to eat from the cart.

You know the answer is B, of course (C might be a decent solution, but it's a little bit like cheating). Now, the way your child handles your answer may depend on the way you've handled all the questions that preceded it. Once you start saying no, your child will start to get used to hearing it. When children are used to hearing it, they are not so upset at not getting what they want. This is not to say they won't pout or complain, but they may not freak out screaming on the floor in front of the angry, tired, judgmental mob in line behind you. (By the way, if your child does happen to freak out, don't give in. Hang in there. You'll be through the line fast enough, and there's not a parent alive who doesn't understand. For those strangers who give you a look, ignore them and feel good in the fact that you are doing the right thing in saying no. Your respect bucket will be a little more full when it's all over.)

Easy... I promise!

You may find it easier to sleep if your newborn is not in the same room with you. They make so much noise with all their little grunts that you may be up all night worrying whether the baby is okay and may not get any sleep at all.

Okay, back to the future. Your child is now three or four. You're at a holiday program and sitting in the audience. The place is packed. The people who camped outside the building the night before got all the good seats and you and your husband are seated separately. Your youngster is bored and hot and does not want to stay put. What do you do?

A. Let him run up and down the aisle to keep busy. People understand that kids can't sit still, right?

B. Ply him with candy or little toys on the floor, keeping

all the people around you from enjoying the show, even though you should be enjoying the show, too.

C. Take the child to the back of the auditorium and hope you'll have better luck seeing the show next year.

By now, you get the picture. Select C and your child will learn that you mean business. Your respect bucket is now so full that when the next situation arrives, your child will listen to your well-respected advice.

Your child is sixteen. She is on her first date. Things go well until it is time to go home and her date tries to make a move that she is not comfortable with. When your daughter comes home and you ask her how it went, what will she do?

A. Say it went great and go right to bed.

B. Tell you what happened.

C. Tell you what happened and ask for your advice.

While B would be great, C would be even better. You can bet that the respect bucket would have to be pretty full in order to get that kind of response. If there were an answer D, it would be that she would tell you what happened, ask for your advice, and take it. Let's not get greedy.

The point in this exercise is not to achieve perfection. Heaven knows, I've failed many times by saying yes when I should have said no because I've been tired or frustrated. The idea is to address the negative behaviors you see with overall consistency (occasional slip-ups are understandable). You should especially be sure to address these situations:

1. Your child is being disrespectful to you.

2. Your child is being disrespectful to someone else.

3. Your child is being destructive.

There will be many tests of your resolve for the demand for respect. One of the pressures that the mothers of the Information Age feel is to be their child's buddy.

In our society, there is much emphasis placed on the Mommy and Me aspect of mothering. Our generation seems to do more things with our children. We get down on the floor and play games with our kids, we exercise with them, and we have group play dates with them. Truth be told, I could never get the hang of those things. Not that I didn't try. I tried to play action figures with my toddler son. I didn't know what to do with Batman, Spiderman, and the X-men. What do they do? What do they say? I didn't know. There were Batcaves and Batboats, Spiderman motorcycles, and Spiderman web gloves. I was clueless. Once I got Batman into the cave, he would just sit there. I knew my son was looking for more from me. Why hadn't I paid more attention to that last episode of the *Batman and Robin* cartoon instead of folding the laundry? I would try to make up a bit of dialogue. "Hey Batman, how are you?" I'd say. "I'm fine, Robin, how are you?" My son looked at me as though I had two heads. Dejected, I would call my mom. "Why don't I have the patience to sit down and play with him?" My mother would say, "Claudine, you are a grown woman. How can you expect to get enjoyment out of the same game an eight-year-old plays?"

I know, I know, we are supposed to be all things to our children and play with them frequently. If you are not particularly creative this way, I advise you to provide the children with a safe place to play and some toys to play with and let them figure it out. The fact that you are nearby will make your children feel secure and happy.

This concept of being around while your children play is an interesting one. My friend tells me that in Spanish this "being around" concept is called "the shadow" or *la sombra*. It means being near as they play but not necessarily playing with them. Being around means your children know you're there if they need you, but that they have the independence and confidence to figure out games, toys, and projects on their own. As they get older it's a concept that will come in handy. They will likely not want to play with you anymore, but they will still want you around. I sometimes make sure that I'm in the same room with my thirteen year old. Even though he may be on the computer while I'm folding laundry, there is always a chance that he might strike up a conversation about something — especially if his sisters aren't around.

Summary

Parenting requires courage, sacrifice, and perseverance. At times it feels like running a marathon. And when you're tired, you stumble. I know what I should do when responding to my children's behavior, but sometimes I'm just too darn tired. So what's a mother to do? I try to get some sleep, pick myself up, and try a little harder next time. I talk to my parents, my husband, my friends, and my coworkers. I try to learn what works and what doesn't work. When I stumble, I don't give up. I keep on trying. Remember, none of these suggestions is easy and they certainly can't be followed flawlessly. Use them as your guidelines and forgive your lapses. Most of all, I wish you luck. It takes a lot of that, too.

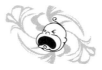

New Mom Glossary

Ok ...so this is not a glossary of technical terms like you might find in other baby books. This is more like a collage of words and phrases that emerge as you go about your daily life as a new mom. Enjoy!

* *at-home mom world* — The new frontier: a world of play dates, strollers, mall walking, new friends, playgrounds, and jungle gyms. Unlike any world you have known before.

* *Baby's Cry 101* — The imaginary course that I should have attended before I brought my baby home. Seriously, I had no idea that the baby would cry so much. I thought something was wrong. That's what you get for doing your research on cable TV.

* *baby schedule* — In some circles this word is taboo. (Did you catch the *Brady Bunch* reference?) In a new mom's world, it is a godsend. Simply stated, a baby schedule is feeding your baby and putting him down for naps at certain times of the day. Embrace it, love it, make it your own!

* *BB* — Before baby — need I say more?

* *Brady Bunch* — A 70s sitcom that I believe encapsulates almost any life lesson. Remember the famous "Bobby runs away from home episode" when Bobby feels that his new stepmother, Carol, won't love him because he is a stepchild? He packs a little suitcase to run away and she meets him at the bottom of the stairs with her own suitcase to run away with him! Are you kidding me? I'm crying as I am typing this! Great stuff. Clearly, I didn't go out much in the 70's as a child.

* *bionic hearing* — The superior hearing a new mother has the moment she returns from the hospital.

* *breast nazi* — Any nurse or lactation specialist who puts on a full-court press for a new mom to breast-feed.

* *counts* — When doing "it" will hopefully result in a pregnancy.

* *demand feeding* — The industry term for feeding a baby whenever he is hungry. OK, I'll bite. How do you know if a baby is hungry? Ahh, here is the problem. Truth is, in the beginning, you don't know when a

baby is hungry — at least I didn't. So for the first few weeks you would be feeding the baby 24/7 — hence my dislike of demand feeding. Come to the light, start a baby schedule.

* *full of soup* — My nana's favorite saying. Same as "full of shit."

* *good baby* — A baby that sleeps a lot and doesn't cry a lot. (I hear they exist but I have never had one of my own.)

* *housewife* — Who knows? The definition of this word evolves with each generation. Suffice to say, a wife who takes care of the house and everything that that entails. Can be a working or nonworking woman. Similar to the Bionic Woman. She has a regular career by day and turns into a superhero type spy when needed.

* *ice pack pads* — Made for new mothers, these may be the best invention next to the epidural. Note: Can also be used after the big event for any injury requiring the use of an ice pack.

* *La sombra* — Spanish for "the shadow." A concept that recommends you stay close by your baby but not in his face so he can learn on his own.

* *mother-guilt* — The guilt all mothers feel if not "doing" for her child and family 100 percent of the time.

* *mommy wars* — The term used to describe the ongoing battle, real or perceived, between the "working" moms and stay-at-home moms. Do I believe it exists? You betcha!

* *new deafness* — The ailment that befalls a husband the moment he returns from the hospital with a newborn.

* *ready* — Our generation's barometer by which we decide to procreate.

* *respect bucket* — A term of measurement, specifically measuring how much respect you have from your children at any given point in time.

* *scary chapters* —Well-meaning but scary information regarding childbirth and what happens after childbirth. These stories are everywhere — in books, in magazines, and within each and every woman who sees you are pregnant. My advice, don't read (or listen to) them unless you have a good reason to.

* *self-actualization* — Maslow's concept of the process by which each person achieves her best self. Kind of like the movie *Groundhog Day* when Bill Murray has to live the same day over and over until he gets it right. Each of us has the right to reach our potential.

* *strange older women* — Complete strangers who will comment on your pregnant self and later, the behavior of your children. Best remedy: politely smile and move on.

* *superman* — The anesthesiologist who administers your epidural.

* *super pads* — Made especially for new mothers, these are the queen of all feminine protection.

* *the talk* — When you finally decide to sit your husband down on the couch and really talk to him about all those issues you've been avoiding before the arrival of the baby. I like to call it the talk when the hairs on the back of his neck stand up. Hopefully, the talk has come prior to the little bundle; however, it is not uncommon to have the talk after the arrival.

* *TLC's A Baby Story* — The Learning Channel is a cable channel that shows real-life experiences. You are no doubt familiar with *A Wedding Story*. You will now graduate to *A Baby Story* and then *Bringing Home Baby*.

* *trying* — Doing "it" in the hopes of making more people.

* *Third child syndrome* — The effect that a third child has on your parenting technique. Once the third child comes along, the things that used to worry you don't worry you so much anymore. "Wanna watch TV, little guy? Knock yourself out." "What's that? You want to have some M&Ms for breakfast? Go for it."

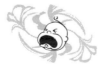

Resources

The truth is you are not going to have much time to read any book from start to finish. You must pick and choose wisely since your time is limited. The resources I include here are in two distinct categories. First are the resources that are so helpful that you just don't want to miss them. The second are the books and websites that you might want to check out when you have a few more minutes in your day.

Read These First!
Books

* *Doctor Spock's Baby and Childcare,* 6th edition, by Benjamin Spock and Michael Rothenberg. This is *the* "baby bible." In this book you will find answers to your baby and childcare questions. It is written succinctly and

with the kindness that a new mother needs. There is absolutely no guilt to be found here. The book contains a great index, making it easy to use as a reference book when you need an answer fast. Amazingly, it can also be read cover to cover.

* *The Mask of Motherhood* by Susan Maushart. My favorite "motherhood" book. If you are looking for honesty about motherhood, you've found it. This is a book you can read by topic as you are experiencing the different phases of motherhood. Ms. Maushart takes the "mask" off of motherhood, revealing the feelings women sometimes hide for fear of being termed a bad mother.

* *Siblings Without Rivalry* by Adele Faber and Elaine Mazlish. This is *the* parenting book, hands down. You may not ever need to read another parenting book — okay, so I'm exaggerating a bit. Truly great insights on how the child's mind works. It is easy to read, simple, and it makes sense with practical applications.

* *On Becoming Babywise*, by Gary Ezzo and Robert Bucknam, M.D. This is a terrific book for the mom who is looking for a flexible feeding and sleep schedule for her baby. The authors include an interesting look at the history behind different parenting techniques. The techniques for the breastfeeding and bottle-feeding mom are detailed and easy to understand.

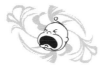

Websites

* *www.Help4NewMoms.com* — My website has all the help a new mom could ask for. Get the advice you need regarding all new mom issues to make your life easier. Check out "true mom confessions" where moms get real about their motherhood experiences. Feel free to contribute your thoughts and ideas for the mothers who will come after you. Download a free baby schedule. Take a break for a laugh or two.

* *www.justmommies.com* — This is a great website for moms who are interested in message boarding. You can sign up to be able to write on the message board or simply read the boards for every imaginable baby and mommy topic. If you are interested in a particular topic and wish to ask a question, the website sends emails with the answers provided by the gals in the group. The women on Just Mommies are very helpful and supportive.

* *www.babycenter.com* — I love this website because it has lots of free stuff for new moms. There is always a calendar or a planner available and fun ways to chart your pregnancy and baby's growth. The site also has a message board. Their helpful, on point articles are some of the best on the Internet.

* *www.cafemom.com* — This is my favorite message boarding website. It has a "social" message boarding feature where you can sign up with a group of friends at the same time to chat by yourselves, much like

Facebook. The site is very slick and has the latest and the greatest graphics, icons, and widgets.

* *www.hybridmom.com* — This is a great website for those of you who consider your self a "Hybrid Mom." You are a mom but you are a bunch of other things, too. The folks at Hybrid Mom understand and have provided a vehicle for you to be heard and to read up on what other women like you are doing. Hybrid Mom has some pretty intense bloggers on staff, as well as a quarterly magazine available nationwide.

* *www.pantley.com*/elizabeth — Elizabeth Pantley's website. She has some great ideas for baby and child care, especially on the topic of sleeping. She offers some free downloadable blank sheets that can be used to write out a schedule. The site offers moms tons of help for their babies and toddlers.

* *www.drspock.com* — You know I am a Dr. Spock fan. What I like most about his site is the great question and answer section for advice at your fingertips. Sometimes you have a specific question and you want an answer fast.

When You're Ready
Books
* *The Inappropriate Baby Book,* by Jennifer Stinson
* *Sippy Cups Are Not For Chardonnay,* by Stephanie Wilder-Taylor
* *The Rookie Mom's Handbook,* by Heather Flett
* *The Colic Chronicles,* by Tara Kompare

* *Mothers Need Time-Outs, Too,* by Susan Callahan
* *Mojomom,* by Amy Tiemann
* *Mommy's High Heel Shoes,* by Kristie Finnan
* *Absolutely Organized,* by Deb Lillard
* *The Second Nine Months,* by Vicki Glembocki
* *Peeing in Peace,* by Beth Feldman
* *Baby Laughs,* by Jenny McCarthy
* *The Feminine Mystique,* by Betty Friedan
* *I Was a Really Good Mom Before I Had Kids,* by Tricia Ashworth and Amy Nobile
* *The Price of Motherhood,* by Ann Crittenden
* *The Prophet,* by Kahil Gibran
* *The Red Tent,* by Anita Diamant
* *The Right To Be Human: A Biography of Abraham Maslow,* by Edward Hoffman

Mom Blogs

* *www.babyonbored.blogspot.com* — Stephanie Wilder-Taylor's mom blog. Taylor blogs honestly and humorously about everything: her life, her twins, her marriage, her doctor's appointments and everything in between. She involves her audience with different contests and questions. Her blog is always entertaining.

* *www.Mom2My6Pack.blogspot.com* — Mother of five shares her life's ups and downs in hysterical posts day after day. She includes pictures of things she finds in her yard or on her roof. Her life is the mirror of so many moms out there that she offers moms a big sigh of relief. I don't know how she does it, but she always makes me laugh.

* *www.mom-101.blogspot.com* — Funny blog filled with real-life mom issues. Liz is a talented writer who knows her audience because she is living motherhood right along with you. You'll enjoy a break in your day with her anecdotes.

* *www.literarymama.com* — Writings by other mothers on all kinds of topics, sometimes very serious. If you are interested in writing yourself, this might be an avenue for you to submit some of your work.

* *www.mojomom.blogspot.com* — Interesting site for mothers and their issues. Amy Tiemann is the author of *Mojomom*. Her blog is terrific and keeps moms informed on the latest issues related to them. She does the work on current affairs so we don't have to. Check out her blog to get informed on the latest and the greatest in politics, new movies, new books, and the media.

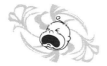

Notes

Chapter Two

1. Dr. Bhavani Shankar Kodali, M.D., "History of childbirth pain relief," http://www.painfreebirthing.com/evolution.htm

2. Stephanie Wilder-Taylor, *Sippy Cups Are Not for Chardonnay* (New York: Simon Spotlight Entertainment, 2006), p.13.

3. Jenny McCarthy, *Baby Laughs* (New York: Penguin Group, 2006), p. 15.

Chapter Four

1. Centers for Disease Control and Prevention, "Provisional Data – National Immunization Survey, 2005 births," http://www.cdc.gov/breastfeeding/data/NIS_data/data_2005.htm

2. Brigham Young University, "New breastfeeding survey study shows most moms quit early," http://byunews.byu.edu/print.aspx?release=archive08/Jul/breastfeed

3. American Academy of Pediatrics, "Breastfeeding and the Use of Human Milk," AAP Policy., http://aappolicy.aapublications.org/cgi/content/full/pediatrics%3b100/6/1035#reference

4. Wilder-Taylor, p. 10.

5. Ask. Dr. Sears, "What attachment parenting is — the 7 baby B's," http://www.askdrsears.com/ht,l/10/T130300.asp

Chapter Six

1. Wilder-Taylor, p. 150.

2. American College of Obstetricians and Gynocologists, "Getting in shape after your baby is born," ACOG. http://www.acog.org/publications/patient_education/bp131.cfm.

3. WebMD,"Get Your Body Back After Pregnancy," http://women.webmed.com/features/get-your-body-back-after-pregnancy?print=true

Chapter Seven

1. Extracted from Dr. Spock's *Baby and Childcare* by Benjamin Spock, M.D., and Michael B Rothenberg, M.D. Copyright 1945, 1946, 1957, 1968, 1976, 1985, 1992 by Benjamin Spock M.D. Reprinted with permission of Pocket Books, a division of Simon & Shuster, Inc. p. 247.

2. Teresa Pitman, "Fear of Spoiling," http://www.todaysparent.com/pregnancybirth/article.jsp?content=3923&page=1

3. Spock and Rothenberg, p.11.

Chapter Eight

1. Spock and Rothenberg, p. 99.

2. Karen Rizzo, "New Mom's Handbook," *Fit Pregnancy*, April-May 2003.

3. Spock and Rothenberg, p. 102.

Chapter Nine

1. U.S. Census Bureau, "Fertility of American Women: June 2004," http://www.census.gov/population/www/scodemo/fertility.html

2. Lee Lusardi Connor, "Guide for Smart Working Moms," http://redbookmag.com/print-this/kids-family/advice/smart-working-moms-guide-hl?click=main_sr

3. BabyCenter"How do I make sure my boss knows I'm working hard if I can't put in long hours?" http://www.babycenter.com/404_how-do-i-make-sure-my-boss-knows-im-working-hard-if-i-cant-p_6118.bc

Chapter Ten

1. Dr. Laura Schlessinger, *The Proper Care and Feeding of Husbands* (New York: HarperCollins, 2004), p. 172.

2. Spock and Rothenberg, p. 17.

Chapter Eleven

1. Ann Crittenden, *The Price of Motherhood* (New York: Henry Holt & Co., 2001), p. 131.

2. Crittenden, 139.

3. Betty Freidan, *The Feminine Mystique* (New York: W. W. Norton and Company, 1964), p.15.

4. Crittenden, p. 138.

Chapter Twelve

1. Susan Maushart, *Wifework*: *What Marriage Really Means for Women* (New York: Bloomsbury, 2003), p. 101.

Chapter Thirteen

1. Abraham H. Maslow, *Toward a Psychology of Being* (New York: D.Van Nostrand Company, 1968)

2. Ibid.

3. Quotations Page, Quotations from Martha Graham, **http://www.quotationspage.com**

Chapter Fourteen

1. Kahil Gibran, *The Prophet* (New York: Alfred A. Knopf, Inc., 1994), p. 17.

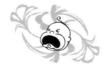

Index

A
adjustment period, 120–121
advice
  from nurses, 18–19
  from strangers, 6
  from *Supernanny,* 88
American College of Obstetrics and Gynecology, 9–10
anesthesia, 9–10, 19–20
asking for help, 100
at-home mom world, *see* stay-at-home moms
attachment parenting, 31

B
BabyCenter, 83
Baby Commandment(s), 56–65
  for burping baby, 63–64
  following, 99
  for giving baby naps, 60–61
  for holding baby during the day, 62–63
  for not bringing baby into your bed, 64–65
  for putting baby down to sleep, 57–59
  for waking baby to feed him/her, 63
Baby Laughs (Jenny McCarthy), 11
baby monitors, 59
baby schedule, 2–3, 66–75
  as basic guideline, 70
  following, 99
  as help for working moms, 83–84
  for jaundiced babies, 42
  natural, 71
  origin of, 71
  for other caregivers, 72–73
  reactions against, 70–72
  rigid, 74
  value of, 68, 74–75
  when breastfeeding, 31
babysitters, finding, 140, 143
bad behavior, addressing, 152, 154, *see also* saying "no"
baskets, organizing with, 131
bathrooms, cleaning, 129
baths, for baby, 43
bed, bringing baby into, 45, 64, 65, 149
bedtime routine, 114